W9-BZY-329

No More
Sleepless Nights

NO MORE SLEEPLESS NIGHTS

· · ● ● ● ● · ·

PETER HAURI, PH.D.

Director
Mayo Clinic Insomnia Program
and Professor of Psychology, Mayo Medical School

SHIRLEY LINDE, PH.D.

WILEY

JOHN WILEY & SONS, INC.

New York   Chichester   Brisbane   Toronto   Singapore

In recognition of the importance of preserving what has been written, it is a policy of John Wiley & Sons, Inc. to have books of enduring value published in the United States printed on acid-free paper, and we exert our best efforts to that end.

This publication is designed to provide accurate and authoritative information in regard to the subject matter covered. It is sold with the understanding that the publisher and authors are not engaged in rendering medical or other professional service. If medical advice or other expert assistance is required, the services of a competent professional person should be sought. The names used for case histories are not patients' real names.

Copyright © 1990, 1991 by Peter Hauri and Shirley Linde.

All rights reserved. Published simultaneously in Canada.

Reproduction or translation of any part of this work beyond that permitted by section 107 or 108 of the 1976 United States Copyright Act without the permission of the copyright owner is unlawful. Requests for permission or further information should be addressed to the Permission Department, John Wiley & Sons, Inc.

Library of Congress Cataloging-in-Publication Data

Hauri, Peter.
    No more sleepless nights / Peter Hauri, Shirley Linde.
      p. cm.
    Includes bibliographical references.
    ISBN 0-471-50770-9   ISBN 0-471-54796-4 (Pbk)
    1. Insomnia—Treatment. I. Linde, Shirley Motter. II. Title.
  RC548.H385 1990   89-22606
  616.8'498—dc20
Printed in the United States of America
10 9 8 7 6 5

To our respective children:
Scott and Bob; Heidi, David, and Kate;
and to our parents

Acknowledgments

The authors wish to thank the following peer reviewers for their contributions during the development of this book:

Philip Westbrook, M.D.
Director, Sleep Disorders Center
Cedars-Sinai Medical Center
Los Angeles, California

Rosalind Cartwright, Ph.D.
Professor and Chairman, Department of Psychology and Social
    Sciences
Rush-Presbyterian-St. Luke's Medical Center
Chicago, Illinois

Ernest Hartmann, M.D.
Director, Sleep Disorders Center
Newton-Wellesley Hospital
Professor of Psychiatry, Tufts University School of Medicine
Boston, Massachusetts

James K. Walsh, Ph.D.
Director, Sleep Disorders Center
Deaconess Hospital
St. Louis, Missouri

Authors' Note

In describing this program, we have a problem with "we," since the entire book was a collaboration between us, but some of the personal and clinical experiences involved only one of us. We ask the reader's indulgence in the occasional lapse from the editorial "we" to the "we" referring to Dr. Hauri and his colleagues at various sleep disorders centers. Dr. Hauri's personal experiences are shown by sections in italic.

We recommend that this program, as any other medical program, should be followed under the approval and guidance of a physician.

Foreword

When Ben Franklin wrote, "But in this world nothing is certain but death and taxes," he might have added insomnia. Certainly, it must be the rare individual who, concerned about death, taxes, or any of the myriad stresses of our lives, has not had difficulty sleeping on occasion. Yet most of us accept a single poor night's sleep because we can identify the cause and know that it will be a transient difficulty. We don't like it, but we can accept it. Unfortunately, there are many people who must face night after night of unsatisfying sleep. This unique book by Doctors Hauri and Linde will help these sufferers of chronic insomnia and will benefit even the person who sleeps poorly only rarely.

The problem of sleeplessness is not just one of discomfort and frustration. While we still do not understand all the reasons that we and so many living things need to sleep, it is clear that sleep is necessary to keep us alert. Sleep loss ultimately will lead to debilitating sleepiness and its sometimes catastrophic effects on judgment and motivation. Thus, this book is critically important and addresses a major health problem.

What makes this book so wonderfully useful is the straightforward, practical, step-by-step approach that the reader can take to help himself or herself overcome the problem of insomnia. Doctor Hauri asks the reader to become his or her own personal scientist—to take specified steps to discover what problem may be causing sleeplessness and then to test the theory by taking certain corrective action. These are not just vague generalities about "relaxing," but specific recommendations for what to do and how to do it.

Doctor Hauri knows that insomnia is a disorder that a patient, given direction, frequently can solve. The direction is given in this book.

The author's credentials are impeccable. Doctor Linde is a well-known science writer. Doctor Hauri is, in my opinion, the world's leading authority on insomnia. He has spent his entire professional career in the scientific study of sleep disorders, specializing in the problems of initiating and maintaining sleep. However, it is not just his ability as a scientist that is critical to this book. He has vast clinical experience in treating patients with insomnia and a unique ability to teach what he has learned.

Together, Doctors Hauri and Linde have teamed up to create a readable, focused, fascinating book that should be read by anyone who has been faced with sleepless nights and knows that it can happen again. Ben Franklin, that wise old lark, told us about "early to bed and early to rise." This book tells us how to spend that time asleep.

Philip R. Westbrook, M.D.
Director, Sleep Disorders Center
Cedars-Sinai Medical Center
Los Angeles, California

Contents

No More
Sleepless Nights

Introduction: Many Suffer, Few Are Treated

You've been there. Everybody has been there at some time in their life. You're worried about something. You're tense, anxious. You go to bed exhausted, but you toss and turn, knowing you need sleep, but you're unable to turn off your worries. You lie awake most of the night, frustrated, your muscles tight, your mind racing—until, exhausted and worn, you fall into troubled, fitful sleep for an hour or two before morning. You are experiencing insomnia.

It may last only this night, but it can last for weeks, months, years, or even a lifetime. It can affect your health, your marriage, your job—every aspect of your life. You stumble through the day at half efficiency, irritable or depressed, dreading the coming night—knowing that, once again, you may be robbed of sleep.

You are not alone.

Many people think that "insomnia" refers only to the severe, chronic sleeplessness that keeps you up all night. It doesn't. It also refers to the occasional sleepless night and to milder forms of poor sleep that might not send you to the doctor, but that rob you of alertness and energy the next day. Insomnia can refer to everyday difficulty in getting to sleep or to problems with waking up in the middle of the night and not being able to get back to sleep.

It is estimated that more than 100 million Americans have occasional sleep problems. About a third of these have some form of chronic insomnia. Millions of others experience unexplained sleepiness in the daytime, nightmares, jerking or cramping of the muscles at night, snoring or gasping for breath, sleepwalking, bedwetting, tooth grinding—the list goes on. This book deals with all the forms of insomnia, both serious and mild.

About 10 million insomniacs suffer enough to consult a physician. People spend millions of dollars on tranquilizers and sleeping pills, looking for help. Recent studies show that one out of every two people has taken sedatives or tranquilizers at some time, and one in five uses them frequently. But pills are not the answer.

Sleep problems occur from infancy to old age, and the incidence increases significantly with age. In fact, in a number of cases, medical advances have been used to prolong a patient's life—then the person must live it through a haze of insomnia and crippling daytime drowsiness.

The A. C. Nielsen Company found that very late into the night—between midnight and 3 A.M.—there are an average of some 20 million Americans up watching television. Many of these people are experiencing insomnia.

Many people—at all ages—are suffering from insomnia, but few are being treated properly. The truth is that in most cases, these victims no longer have to suffer night after night.

Only 25 years ago, there wasn't much we could do for insomnia. We knew almost nothing about it, nor about sleeping pills. For many years, we didn't know that withdrawing from sleeping pills could cause a serious worsening of insomnia or that sleeping pills could slow down respiration. Therefore, these pills were handed out rather freely.

Later, there was an explosion in knowledge about sleep and its disorders. To disseminate the new information, the U.S. Surgeon General's office—along with various medical organizations, pharmaceutical companies, and consumers' groups—launched Project Sleep, a program to inform physicians and the public about sleep disorders. While still more needs to be done, the average physician today is much more knowledgeable than most physicians were 25 years ago.

The problem is that not enough of this information is reaching the general public. There are many things we have learned in recent years that insomniacs could do for themselves if they had the information.

That's why we are writing this book. We want to get the message out, so that people will know about the latest professional help available to them, as well as learning about the many things they can do for themselves if they have problems sleeping. There *is* hope.

Poor Sleep May Be Hazardous to Your Health

"Of all the medical problems today, few are as wide-ranging and as little understood as sleep disorders," says the American Sleep Disorders Association (the major national organization that includes all the major sleep disorders centers, as well as professionals specializing in sleep problems). This prestigious group points out that the ramifications of insomnia and other sleep disorders are much greater than most people realize.

For example, chronic insomniacs not only have miserable nights, but often feel so exhausted at work that productivity suffers. Often, they are so worn out after work that they give up leisure activities and social engagements, and the quality of their lives severely deteriorates. A study of 3,000 New England high-school students showed that 30 percent fell asleep in school at least once a week.

Sleep loss accumulates, and many people carry a dangerously large sleep debt, often unknowingly. A person with a big sleep debt is slower to recover from stress and is much more vulnerable to infections and other illnesses and to the effects of alcohol. As the sleep debt grows, the pressure to sleep while on the job or on the road increases.

How often is this a factor when drivers veer off the road, workers record the wrong numbers, or technicians push the wrong buttons? Many air and train crashes, as well as industrial accidents (including several nuclear power plant incidents), appear to have involved sleep loss or upsets in sleep rhythms. In some of these accidents, it seems that someone literally was asleep at the switch.

The more we learn about sleep, the more we realize just how important sleep is to our general health—indeed, to the quality of our entire lives.

Sleep Study—A New Frontier

The systematic study of sleep is relatively new—very little sleep research was done until 1953. Then, at the University of Chicago, Dr. Nathaniel Kleitman first noticed that rapid eye movements occurred occasionally during sleep. Dr. Kleitman worked with a young graduate student, Eugene Aserinsky, to study these eye movements. They taped electrodes near volunteers' eyes and were astonished to learn that the rapid eye movements not only occurred in everybody they tested, but also occurred about every 90 minutes during sleep. A sophomore medical student, William Dement, joined Dr. Kleitman's team and wondered if the sleeping person's eyes might be looking at something, such as a dream. So they started waking sleepers during these times and found that, sure enough, people were usually dreaming.

From these experiments, the researchers realized that there were two distinct types of sleep—a quiet type and an active type with dreaming. It was this breakthrough that created excitement about sleep research. The researchers began to monitor the sleep of thousands of people of all ages throughout the night. They even studied some people who were blind, including the famous pianist, George Shearing. They found that Shearing and other people who had been blind from birth did not have rapid eye movements, but did display the same brain-wave patterns during dreaming—and dreamed of sounds instead of sights.

· · · ● ● · · ·

It was 1960 when I joined the University of Chicago team as a graduate student, working as an assistant to Dr. Allen Rechtschaffen. Those were heady times! Just a month before I came aboard, Dr. Rechtschaffen had called all the world's sleep researchers that he knew to Chicago for a sleep conference. Almost all of them had come—from the United States, Canada, England, France, and Italy—all 12 of them! Just a year later, at the second sleep conference in Chicago, there were about 25 of us, and five years later there were close to 300. The excitement about sleep research was growing.

For the first ten years, almost all work in the sleep field was in research, not in treatment. During the 1960s, we simply did not know enough to treat patients with sleep problems. Then, in the late 1960s, Dr. Anthony Kales at UCLA started a sleep disorders center for patients. Dr. Dement at Stanford opened one not much later, and in 1971, I opened a center at Dartmouth in New Hampshire. These centers showed that, indeed, you can help many patients when you study them in the lab. The idea caught on like wildfire, and now almost every major medical center in the United States has a sleep disorders center.

The fast growth of these centers had some problems, too—some unqualified persons opened centers. In 1975, I called together a conference to talk about ways to evaluate skills and monitor standards of centers. The American Sleep Disorders Association was born at that meeting, and the maintenance of high professional standards is still its main goal.

· · · ● ● ● · ·

In the last ten years, more sleep disorders centers have opened, and 1990 found more than 125 fully accredited centers in hospitals, medical schools, and clinics. Many more are planned.

A few years ago, there were only a handful of scientists specializing in sleep disorders. Now, there are more than 1,200 somnologists (the scientific name for specialists who study and treat sleep disorders) in the United States.

But progress often moves slowly. It is unfortunately true that many people still suffer from poor sleep, but don't know that there is much that can help them. We don't want that to be true any longer, and that is why we wrote this book for all those who have problems with insomnia and other poor sleep.

What This Program Will Give You

In this book, we will tell you about the latest, important research on sleep. We will tell you step by step about the programs used at major sleep disorders centers and how patients' disorders are investigated, diagnosed, and treated there. We'll also give you practical advice about your own sleep fitness, including things you can do at home to help yourself conquer insomnia or other sleep problems.

All this information will be given in simple and practical terms. We will explain each approach to good sleep with easy-to-follow guidelines. This should make it as easy as possible for you to choose the techniques that are best for your own particular situation, so that you can successfully find your own path to sleeping well.

There is one philosophy shared by all doctors at sleep disorders centers: Insomnia is not a disease; it is a symptom. The first thing you have to do is find out what kind of insomnia you have and what is causing it. Insomnia is like pain: You can relieve it with a pill for a little while, but pills won't help in the long run. If you have chronic pain, you can't just take more pills indefinitely. But that's what many people, and their doctors, do with insomnia. Instead of finding out what is causing the insomnia, they treat it symptomatically with sleeping pills.

Because there are different kinds of insomnia, and different causes for them, there is no one program for everyone with insomnia. In fact, when it comes to recommendations, what is good for one kind of insomnia may very well be bad for another. Our program will help you find the underlying cause of your particular problem and then the best treatment for it.

Often, insomnia is caused by stress, but there are many other causes also. Insomnia may occur because you have a daily sleep-wake rhythm that doesn't match the world's 24-hour cycle. Or you may have depression, anxiety, or other psychological problems causing the insomnia. Or there may be medical causes—a hormone upset, something causing pain, or even a reaction to a medication you are taking. Insomnia can even be caused by an allergy, your diet, smoking, or drinking too much alcohol before you go to bed.

It may be that your own body is waking you up in the middle of the night—with twitching of your legs or breathing problems. Or you may be getting sleep, but it's nonrestorative sleep (you sleep long enough, but your sleep is such that you don't get anything out of it). Or you may simply have some bad sleeping habits—bad sleep hygiene.

When a survey on sleep was done by the Gallup Organization, people cited such reasons for their difficulty in sleeping as thinking over problems, being unable to relax, muscle or joint aches, dreams, noise, a light, or someone else's snoring. But 85 percent said they had never discussed their sleeping difficulties with a doctor, even though a high percentage felt that their problem was severe. You may get help for any of these problems from the program in this book.

Our program consists of many different recommendations and approaches. Each insomnia is different. Some facets of the program you read in the book will apply to you; other things will not. The strength of our program lies in the fact that we give you a scientific method by which you can evaluate what will, and what will not, help in your own case. Using this method, by the time you finish this book you should have a highly personalized treatment program with which to combat your sleep problem, one that is different from anybody else's who has read the book.

In this program, we'll help you learn the most likely causes of your own sleeping problem and what to do about those causes. You will become your own sleep therapist, analyzing your own particular situation and trying several parts of the program for a week or two—then, if that doesn't work, going on to try something else.

The program includes tests and questionnaires to evaluate your sleep history and your sleep lifestyle and will tell you how to set up Sleep Logs like those used in the leading sleep disorders centers. It will guide you through specific steps on how to use the latest sleep center techniques at home yourself, including new sleep-promoting habits, relaxation techniques, stress management, diet, and exercise— all designed to guide you on the way to better sleep. The program will tell you how to use the new techniques of light therapy and chronotherapy to reset a sleep clock that could be out of sync, and even gives you new techniques for counteracting sleep problems due to shift work, jet lag, and winter depression. And, importantly, the program will tell you step by step how to kick the sleeping pill habit or, if you can't kick it, how to know when you might need further help.

The program will take patience, time, and persistence. But if you follow the program carefully, there is an excellent likelihood that you'll be sleeping much better when you are finished.

The Program's Results

Using the program approach described in this book, results with patients have been excellent. Of the patients who have used the program—patients so bothered by their insomnia that they have gone beyond their own personal physicians to the sleep center—at least four out of five have been helped. After analyzing a set of questions sent to them and keeping a Sleep Log (page 42), they spend about an hour and a half in a discussion of what has been found in relation to their specific problem and what should be tried to solve it.

When we contact people first at one month and then at three months after they begin the program, about 80 percent of those who follow the recommendations report that their sleep is "remarkably better"! These patients report that after being on the program, their sleep is sounder and more restful. Most of them no longer even worry about their sleep because, in fact, insomnia usually has ceased to be a problem in their lives.

We want you to have the same results.

We welcome you to this program to help solve *your* sleep problem, and we wish you success—so that you, too, can look forward to much better nights and more fulfilled days.

···1···

The Facts About Sleep

Sleep is interwoven with every facet of daily life. It affects our health and well-being, our moods and behavior, our energy and emotions, our marriages and jobs, our very sanity and happiness.

Poets and philosophers have written about sleep. Painters and sculptors, from the Renaissance to Picasso, have made it part of art.

All of us do it nearly every night of our lives (about a third of the human lifetime is spent in sleep), yet most of us know little about it.

People used to think of sleep as a time of quiet, of inactivity. But during sleep, a lot of complex activity occurs both in the brain and in the body. Sleeping doesn't turn off your body systems; in fact, some of them are more turned on during sleep than they are during wakefulness. Indeed, there are some medical disorders that occur only during sleep and go away when you are awake. This idea is so new that some medical textbooks only a few years old are out of date because they haven't incorporated this new concept.

What is sleep? What controls this universal cycle that is as natural as night following day? Why does one person "sleep like a log" and another toss and turn all night?

There are many questions. Before we present the specific steps of the program, we want to explore some of the questions frequently asked of sleep experts. The answers will give you some of the facts that have been learned in research laboratories and may help you separate sleep facts from fiction.

How Much Sleep Do You Really Need?

This is the first question that everybody asks.

The answer: The amount of sleep that people need varies tremendously. There is no "normal" amount. Different people need different amounts of sleep.

But the amount that any one person needs is amazingly constant. Although you may sleep longer one night than another, depending on circumstances, the number of hours you sleep over a week or a month usually averages out very much the same—one week usually falls within *one-half hour* of another week.

Eight hours of sleep a night is the usual quoted average, although seven to seven and a half hours is in reality a more usual estimate. Even that is only an average and has nothing to do with what's good or bad. A good night's sleep can range from less than three hours to more than ten.

About 150 years ago, before Thomas Edison developed the electric light, our entire society slept about an hour longer, a little more than eight hours. Some people say it hasn't hurt us any to stay up longer with the electric light, that all we do is sleep a little more soundly and deeply. Other people say that the frenetic pace of our modern living has to do with Edison's giving us light and leading us to stay up longer than we really should.

We don't expect everybody in the world to wear the same size shoes, but somehow people think that we should all sleep the same length of time. We worry if someone doesn't sleep the magic eight hours, and if they need more sleep, we call them lazy. But two people out of every ten (slightly more in men) sleep less than six hours each night, according to the National Health Center for Statistics. And about one in ten sleeps nine hours or more a night.

Sleep researchers call people who sleep six hours or less *short sleepers* and people who sleep nine hours or more *long sleepers*. Napoleon and Edison were both short sleepers, reported to get only four to six hours a night. Einstein, on the other hand, was a long sleeper, as many other creative people in science and the arts have been.

Some people seem to get by on very little sleep. When two sleep researchers put an ad in a newspaper asking for people who slept only a few hours each night, they found a 54-year-old executive and a 30-year-old draftsman, who both said they slept only about three hours a night. A week in the sleep lab confirmed it. Both said that they just didn't feel they needed more sleep.

One 70-year-old nurse was sent to the laboratory for evaluation because she slept so little. She slept only a little more than an hour per night when she was monitored for five nights in the lab. She took no naps during the day and said she didn't feel tired. In fact, she didn't understand why other people wasted so much time sleeping. She said she had averaged only one hour of sleep a night since childhood.

Another patient, a 71-year-old woman, was sent to the sleep clinic at Dartmouth because she had never slept more than three hours a night through her entire adult life. She felt well during the day, still cross-country skied every day in the winter, hiked frequently during the summer, and was politically active in her town. A checkup at the sleep center showed that her sleep was exceptionally sound, and, indeed, she was quite healthy and getting enough sleep.

A well-known physicist, on the other hand, needs ten hours of sleep each night. If he gets only eight hours, he has great difficulty concentrating. He says he feels like he has a tight band around his head and that he is so foggy he can't do his research. If he gets ten hours of sleep, he's fine.

So how much sleep you need varies from person to person.

Individuals also can have different sleep needs at different times. They may need more sleep in times of stress, during depression or grief, or during times of increased mental effort. The authors spent more time in bed than usual while writing this book, for example. Some women sleep more during premenstrual periods. Less sleep may be needed during times when things are going especially well for a person.

Does Sleep Change with Age?

It was once thought that you needed more sleep as you get older. Now we know that once you reach adulthood, you require about the same amount of sleep at all ages.

However, the *pattern* of sleep does change. The older person often sleeps more lightly. As the body ages, the quality of sleep usually deteriorates—sleep becomes less efficient, lighter, and less restful. There is a gradual decrease in delta sleep (the deepest sleep, most associated with growth and bodily recovery) throughout life. By around age 50 for men and 60 for women, there is much less of the deep delta sleep, sometimes none, so that at these ages and older, people are more easily aroused by noises or other outside factors that younger people might sleep through.

Although the length of sleep time in a healthy person does not change from about age 20 to about age 75, the incidence of sleep problems does increase. Sleep is more disturbed and there is sleep time lost because of interruptions. This means that you may spend more time in bed and may think you sleep longer, but your sleep frequently is interrupted by brief periods of wakefulness. Some older people have hundreds of short awakenings at night, lasting 15 seconds or less. Sometimes, these little awakenings give you the impression that you've been awake all night, even though you haven't been. Sometimes, just knowing that this is a possibility helps you to be more relaxed about your sleep. Older persons also may take more naps during the day, which gives them even more wakefulness at night.

Remember, the amount and quality of your sleep are usually normal if it seems so to you and if your daytime efficiency and alertness are not decreased.

What About Sleep in Children?

Newborn infants sleep an average of 16-1/2 hours daily and by six months usually average about 14 hours. At age 2 the average sleep time is 12-1/2 hours; 1-1/2 hours of nap time and 11 hours at night. By age 6 most children no longer need naps, and sleep time is reduced to about 11 hours. Sleep time of the 10-year-old averages 10 hours, and from ages 15 to 19 it averages around 7-1/2 to 8-1/2 hours. The variations in amount of sleep taken by a child from day to day may be large, but, as in adults, the weekly or monthly averages for the same child are surprisingly consistent.

Remember, however, that the averages cited here may be quite meaningless for an individual child. For example, Peter's son, who is about two years younger than Peter's older daughter, slept less than his sister did throughout childhood. For awhile, Peter was concerned that he got so much less sleep than she did, but it does not seem to have hurt him. So if your child does not fit these averages, there is no need to worry, as long as the child functions well and does not fall asleep during the day. If a child has to be stimulated all the time and then falls asleep when watching TV or doing something else quiet, then that child is not getting enough sleep.

What Really Happens in Sleep?

When you are asleep, the kind of electroencephalographic (EEG) waves your brain is producing differs from those made when you are awake. When you're awake, the brain makes either very small, fast waves or alpha waves (ten cycles per second); when you are asleep, it makes slower and bigger waves, the delta and theta waves. The reason: When you are awake, each nerve cell in your brain fires individually. What is being recorded on the EEG is the average of millions of nerve cells, as they fire, their positive and negative electrical charges cancel each other out, and the average approaches zero. That's why the waves are very small and the fluctuations from positive to negative are very fast. When you're asleep, more of the nerve cells start working together and, like a bunch of feet all tapping to the same beat, they discharge at the same time, which makes the waves slower and larger.

There are two kinds of sleep: REM sleep and non-REM sleep (pronounced "non-rem" and usually written NREM). NREM sleep is normal, orthodox sleep; REM sleep is dreaming sleep.

REM stands for *rapid eye movement*, because our eyes move rapidly during that stage. We look around in our dreams. Indeed, without any instruments, you can tell whether a person is dreaming simply by watching the closed eyes. If the bulge of the eyeball underneath the closed eyelids moves rapidly, the person is in REM sleep. Watch for at least 30 seconds or so, because sometimes there are pauses between groups of eye movements.

Interestingly, the brain does not seem to know that we are dreaming, but still gives commands to our muscles to carry out the actions we dream about. Luckily, just before dreaming starts, a nucleus of nerve cells deep within the brainstem relaxes all our muscles so deeply that they are practically paralyzed. During dreaming, our brain's commands to move these muscles result only in very little movements, and this lets us sleep through our dreams. You might have seen these little twitches in cats or dogs as they dream.

In research animals, it is possible to block out the nucleus that inhibits muscle tension during REM sleep. These animals then carry out their dreams. Although their eyes are closed, they crouch, scratch, hiss, and fight. A similar phenomenon occurs in some people in whom the inhibitory nerve cells are not functioning properly. They may move violently during their dreams, bang on the pillow, fling themselves out of bed, and occasionally hurt themselves. This is called *REM behavior disorder*, and it can be treated.

In most people, REM sleep occurs about every 90 minutes throughout the night (about 60-minute intervals in infants). The first REM period of the night is very short, maybe 5 minutes, the second is about 10 minutes, and the third is maybe 15 minutes. The final dream of the night usually lasts 30 minutes, but sometimes lasts an hour. Everybody dreams several times each night. If you slept about six hours last night, you can be sure you had about four dreams. Most dreams are forgotten, however, unless you wake up from them.

On the other hand, NREM sleep, the nondream sleep, comes in two variations—the most frequent type, called stage 2, and the much deeper version, called delta sleep (or stages 3 and 4). There is some thinking during NREM sleep, but it usually is simple and fragmented.

There also is a transition phase between waking and sleeping, when some parts of the brain are asleep while others are not. This is called stage 1 sleep.

Going to sleep is like going down a stairway. You start going down into stage 1 sleep for half a minute to several minutes, with your thoughts drifting, but you don't feel asleep. Then you go down the stairway some more to stage 2, and your brain starts putting out waves with characteristic patterns called *sleep spindles* and *K-complexes*. Then, you go into deep stage 3 and 4 delta sleep.

Sleep specialists call the time to the end of the first REM sleep the *first sleep cycle,* and the time from then to the end of the second REM sleep the *second sleep cycle*. There are four to six sleep cycles per night, depending on how long you sleep. Usually, the changes between sleep stages are gradual, with one stage blending into the next as you gradually move up and down the stairway. In the last part of the night, there usually is no deep delta sleep at all.

Stage 1, although it is called "sleep," is worth hardly anything in terms of its recovery value. Sleep researchers continue to debate the value of the other stages of sleep. Delta sleep generally appears to be the main kind of sleep that allows the body to recover. If you take away delta sleep, you often wake up with a feeling of malaise; though

HUMAN SLEEP STAGES

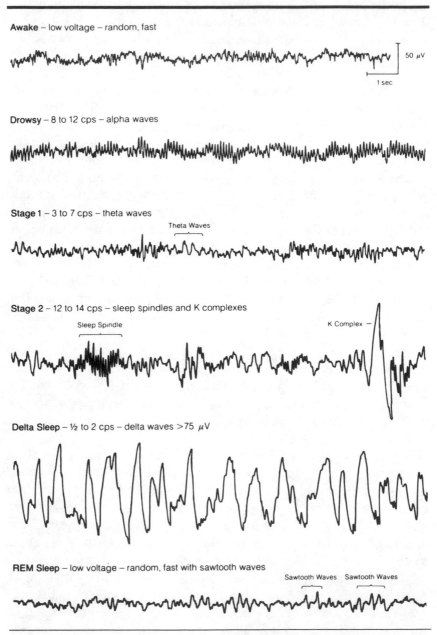

Awake – low voltage – random, fast

50 μV

1 sec

Drowsy – 8 to 12 cps – alpha waves

Stage 1 – 3 to 7 cps – theta waves

Theta Waves

Stage 2 – 12 to 14 cps – sleep spindles and K complexes

Sleep Spindle   K Complex –

Delta Sleep – ½ to 2 cps – delta waves >75 μV

REM Sleep – low voltage – random, fast with sawtooth waves

Sawtooth Waves   Sawtooth Waves

Source: Peter Hauri, *Current Concepts, The Sleep Disorders*, Upjohn, Kalamazoo, Michigan, 1982, p. 7.

Typical Sleep Pattern of a Young Human Adult

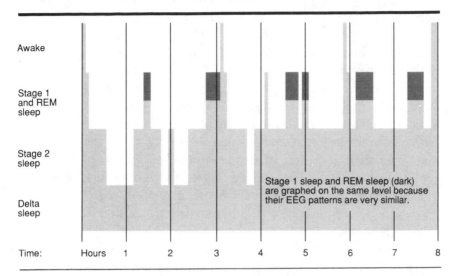

Awake

Stage 1 and REM sleep

Stage 2 sleep

Delta sleep

Stage 1 sleep and REM sleep (dark) are graphed on the same level because their EEG patterns are very similar.

Time: Hours 1 2 3 4 5 6 7 8

nothing in the body is "broken," nothing seems to function right. Stage 2 sleep seems to be a less intense form of delta sleep and, like delta sleep, is concerned mainly with body recovery. On the other hand, REM sleep seems to be more involved with mental recovery. If you don't have REM sleep, it's harder to make sense out of your life.

These are very fine points still debated among sleep researchers. The important thing is not what stages of sleep you're having, but the total amount and quality of sleep you get. It is important that you not have much stage 1 sleep and that your sleep be continuous, not fragmented with awakenings. That's why most sleep clinicians are more concerned that you sleep well than whether the sleep is this or that particular stage.

A lot is going on in the rest of your body in addition to the activity in your brain. During the first one and a half hours or so of sleep, there is a large decrease in heart and respiratory rate and a small drop in blood pressure; after this, there is a further gradual decline in these rates. The lowest levels of heart and respiratory rate, blood pressure, and core temperature occur about an hour before we wake up.

Superimposed on this decline are *increases* in heart and respiratory rate and blood pressure during REM sleep. In fact, heart rate, blood pressure, and respiration sometimes can fluctuate wildly during dreams, possibly accounting for heart attacks and strokes that happen during sleep.

Another interesting fact has to do with blood flow. During delta sleep, when body recovery takes place, most of your blood is directed to the muscles. Although the brain can think during delta sleep, this thinking is sparse and fragmented, since without much blood, the brain barely holds onto a thought. During REM sleep, as our brain wakes up and starts thinking more intensely and dreaming, more blood flow goes into the brain and less goes into the body. Estimates are that as much as a quarter of all blood circulating during REM sleep goes through the brain. Presumably, this increased blood flow is needed to support the increased brain activity during dreaming.

Hormone secretion also is active during sleep, including release of growth hormone. In fact, at the onset of delta sleep, there is the largest spurt of growth hormone in the entire 24-hour cycle. This hormone is used not just for growing, but also for repair of tissue.

What About Sexual Reactions During Sleep?

Both men and women experience sexual reactions during sleep. Men, without knowing it, usually experience an erection during REM periods of sleep (about every 90 minutes). The arousal seems to occur in all males: infants, middle-aged men, men in their 70s and 80s, and even some men who appear to be impotent during waking hours.

Erections seem to occur no matter what the dream is about, even if there is no sexual activity in the dream. Occasionally, an erection is lost suddenly during a dream; typically, this has been found to be associated with an experience of anxiety or injury occurring in the dream.

We use this normal, REM-related erection reflex in sleep laboratories to measure whether male impotence is psychogenic or organic.

As usual, less data exists on sexuality in women, but a few experiments show that women also seem to experience periods of excitation during sleep. Studies show erection of the clitoris and an increase in blood supply to the vaginal area occurring at the same REM intervals during the night.

Why Do Some People Sleep Better Than Others?

The sleep-wake system is extremely complex. It's not just one center or one nucleus, but a whole group of little nerve centers strung from the very lowest parts of the brain and up the brainstem to the forebrain. There appear to be two systems: one pushing arousal, the other pushing sleep. Both are active all the time, and they interact. Whether you sleep or not depends on which of the two is dominant at a certain time. Muscle activity, anxiety, intensive thinking, noise, light, or other stimuli all strengthen the arousal system.

Typically, the arousal system is the stronger of the two. However, its strength decreases naturally after we have been awake for awhile, say 16 hours, or when there is a lack of stimulation. This is why when we want to sleep we seek the quiet of the bedroom, the darkness of closed eyes, and a soft surface to lie on. However, when your mind is preoccupied with some issue or when your body sends out pain stimuli, arousal remains high and the weaker sleep system is not able to overcome the arousal system.

It is natural that in a system as complex as our sleep-wake system, not everybody is equally endowed, just as some are taller and others shorter. The weaker your sleep system (or the stronger your awake system), the more careful you have to be with your sleep.

Often, you can trace strong and weak sleep systems through families. Sometimes, patients will say that their mother or grandmother couldn't sleep. However, just the fact that you can trace insomnia through a family doesn't necessarily mean that it is genetic; it also is possible that the family may be made up of some chronic worriers who fret about every family member's sleep habits, making them overly concerned about their own sleep.

What about Dream Time?

Long sleepers have much more REM sleep than do short sleepers. A very short sleeper typically has a long delta stage of sleep, then a 5-minute REM dream period, lots more delta sleep, then a 10-minute REM period—and that's all the REM sleep for the entire night. The long-sleeping person has five to seven REM dream periods, one every 90 minutes all through the night. Toward morning, the periods get much longer, up to an hour per dream. So a long sleeper may have two to three hours of REM sleep per night, while a short sleeper may get only 15 minutes. This does not seem to hurt the short sleeper.

In some of the early research performed on sleep and dreams, researchers would watch an EEG to tell when sleepers started dreaming, then would wake subjects during the first moments of each dream to prevent them from dreaming. After four or five nights of dream deprivation, volunteers seemed anxious, irritable, and unable to concentrate.

Because of these early studies, it was thought that dream deprivation would cause people to become psychotic. While this has not been confirn.ed, it has been shown that people who have been REM-deprived for a number of nights are more anxious, more agitated, and less controlled (apparently more at the mercy of their primary drives, such as eating uncontrollably). This also can be shown with animals. REM-deprived cats pace more and eat more; after REM deprivation, male cats will mount almost anything that looks like a female, including wooden blocks.

When dreaming is greatly reduced, on the following nights your dreaming sleep starts sooner and lasts much longer, consuming a greater percentage of total sleep time than normally. The dreams also are more intense and sometimes are more bizarre. Apparently, you are making up for lost dream time.

Indeed, not only do we have more REM on nights after we have been deprived of REM dream time, it also has been shown that some of us can start to dream in NREM sleep if we are deprived of REM sleep.

What Happens When You Don't Get Enough Sleep?

Missing one night's sleep is not that bad for your body. If you are giving a speech the next morning, starting a new job, catching a plane, or starting a vacation, it is only natural to have difficulties with sleeping on the previous night. The excitement of the next day's activities almost always counteracts any effects of the loss of sleep.

The main effect of a poor night's sleep, or even two or three, is that you just get very sleepy. You also lose motivation for doing work or anything else but sleeping; it is difficult to pay attention to tasks, especially if they are boring; and your reaction time is somewhat slowed. Monotonous activities such as driving can be risky. So there are some effects, but they usually aren't critical.

For most jobs, performance is not affected by one night's lost sleep. However, making crucial judgments or doing creative thinking can be more difficult, and if a job is extremely boring, there is a decrease in performance even after the loss of just two hours of sleep on one night. Dr. R. Wilkinson, of Cambridge, England, showed this by working with army recruits. He had them do some very boring work—such as crossing out the letter A in a series of words—for many hours a day after losing different amounts of sleep. Even.a loss of only two hours of sleep had an effect. But most of our tasks aren't so boring and, especially in an emergency, adrenalin keeps us going efficiently the next day and makes up for lost sleep.

If you are forced to engage in an activity such as driving after sleep deprivation, you are in much more danger than usual because you are not as attentive or as careful in your judgment, and you might doze off.

When spending an entirely sleepless night—because of an emergency, for example—we may feel most sleepy around the "trough" of the 24-hour cycle, around 4 or 5 in the morning. Then, if we continue to stay awake, we usually get a second wind at about 8, 9, or 10 in the morning and function relatively well again during that day.

Missing sleep on a chronic basis may be a different story. After several nights without sleep, performance does go down, and you have more trouble concentrating and remembering numbers.

In 1959, a disc jockey named Peter Tripp went without sleep for 200 hours to raise money for the March of Dimes. After about five days without sleep, he began to experience hallucinations—believing that somebody's tweed suit was made of worms and that flames were coming out of a drawer. He managed to do his daytime broadcast, but felt that he was in danger at night. After 200 hours of sleeplessness, he slept for 13 hours and was essentially back to normal. However, he reported slight feelings of depression for several months.

In 1964, Randy Gardner, a 17-year-old high-school senior, tried to establish a new record of 260 sleepless hours as a project in his local science fair. He became irritable after about the fourth day, but he retained many skills—after 230 hours of sleep loss, he still was able to hold his own on a pinball machine with sleep researcher Dr. William

C. Dement, director of the Sleep Disorders Center at Stanford University.

Several laboratory experiments have involved sleep deprivation for long periods. It was found that a person's mood deteriorates first— joy disappears—and the person becomes *very* sleepy and grim. After about two or three days, most people start having minisleeps, little lapses of attention when the brain goes to sleep for only five or ten seconds and wakes right up again. By about five days, these minisleeps become longer and more numerous. By ten or eleven days, the minisleeps are so numerous and so mixed with wakefulness that you can't tell whether you are awake or asleep. You can talk, and in the middle of talking have two or three slow waves of sleep. You can walk, and from one step to the next you might catch a second of sleep.

If you are given a task to do yourself, such as adding a column of numbers, the minisleeps may occur without your being aware of them. However, if you are given a paced task—for example, if someone calls out numbers to you that you have to add—you may make many mistakes, because for the few seconds of minisleep, you don't hear the numbers.

Many adults obtain less than optimal sleep, and some have a sizable sleep debt. Like gamblers playing with borrowed money, many sleep-deprived persons live in the red of lost sleep, often compromising their responsibilities at their jobs, sometimes using drugs for temporary energy. Most employees, even in crucial jobs, are forced to keep going all day no matter how fatigued they are. What if such sleep-deprived persons are dealing with the safety of an airplane? What if they are driving a semitrailer down a crowded highway? What if they are making a military decision pivotal to war or peace?

Small sleep losses, built up day after day, can be cumulative. Soon, the chronic loss of sleep can cause lapse of attention, inability to respond, slow thinking, impaired memory, erratic behavior, and irritability. Mental functions decline and judgment fades, with results serious enough to be a danger to the person—and to society, especially when critical decisions are being made, vehicles are being driven, or dangerous machinery is being used. In the sleep centers, we often find people who think they have some serious mental or physical disease when they simply do not allow themselves enough time to sleep.

Sometimes, you have to give up sleep out of sheer necessity—to complete a job that must be done. But don't do it on a regular basis without letting yourself catch up.

You don't have to catch up, by the way, on all the sleep that you have missed. If you have been totally deprived of sleep for about ten days, you will probably sleep for 14 or 18 hours per day for about three days and then go back to your normal schedule.

···· 2 ····

What Kind of Insomniac
Are You?

Some people can't fall asleep, others can't stay asleep. There can even be problems when your sleep is interrupted constantly—brief awakenings that you may not be aware of can prevent much of the good that sleep usually accomplishes.

Author Jacqueline Susann was described as an example of the unable-to-go-to-sleep type of insomniac, spending many late nights on the telephone with other insomniac friends. Benjamin Franklin exemplified the middle-of-the-night-awakening kind of insomniac. He believed that his problem was a rumpled bed, so he bought a second bed—whenever he awoke in the middle of the night, he simply crawled from the bed he was in to the neatly made second bed to complete his night's sleep.

Other famous insomniacs include Napolean Bonaparte, Irving Berlin, Winston Churchill, Charles Dickens, James Thurber, Cary Grant, Dorothy Kilgallen, Oscar Levant, and Marilyn Monroe. You need not feel alone.

The Kinds of Insomnia

To ask yourself what kind of insomniac you are, you first must understand what kind of insomnias exist. Various scientific groups classify insomnia in different ways. One system divides insomniacs into (1) people who can't fall asleep when they go to bed, and (2) people who fall asleep readily but can't stay asleep.

A second system is based on how long the insomnia lasts. It classifies insomnia as *transient insomnia* if it lasts just one to three nights and *short term insomnia* if it lasts from three nights to three weeks and then disappears. *Chronic insomnia* lasts more than three weeks.

A classification system that is used at some sleep disorders centers sorts the causes of insomnia into four main categories:

- Insomnias associated with psychological problems
- Insomnias associated with medical problems
- Insomnias due to lifestyle
- Insomnias caused by poor sleep habits

Evaluating Your Own Insomnia

If you are tossing and turning at night, not getting the kind of sleep you want to have, how can you find the particular set of circumstances that is causing your special insomnia?

If you were a participant in our program, your first diagnostic interview would take between about 40 and 90 minutes. This interview is specifically designed to establish what kind of problem you have and, if you are an insomniac, what kind of insomniac you are.

We are going to give you a self-evaluation procedure that follows the same method in a do-it-yourself version. First, answer the questions in the Sleep History Analysis and other questionnaires in this chapter. The questions and their answers will give you some hunches to follow in learning exactly what is really causing your poor sleep and will help you choose which guidelines to concentrate on in following the various steps of the program.

You may want to write down the questions and your answers in a notebook to have with the Sleep Logs you are going to learn to keep. If you go to a physician or a sleep center for further help, the answers to these questions also will be helpful there.

In the analysis, be open-minded about the possibilities. Getting to the real cause of your problem is essential to the success of the program.

Sleep History Analysis

Now go to page 24 and answer the questions of the Sleep History Analysis. The answers to the first seven questions define the amount

Sleep History Analysis

1. What time do you usually go to bed and get up on weekdays?
2. What time do you usually go to bed and get up on weekends?
3. Do you keep a fairly regular sleep schedule?
4. If you could set your own schedule, when would you go to bed and when would you get up?
5. How long does it usually take for you to fall asleep? Do you have trouble getting to sleep?
6. How often do you wake up during the night? Do you usually have trouble getting back to sleep?
7. How many hours, on the average, do you actually sleep?
8. Do you often feel exhausted during the day because of lack of sleep? Does your excessive sleepiness often interfere with your work or your social life?
9. Have you ever had an accident or near-accident because of sleepiness from not being able to sleep the night before?
10. Do you usually nap during the day? How long, on the average?
11. Do you do shift work?
12. Are you often bothered by waking up earlier than you want to and not being able to get back to sleep?
13. When did your primary difficulty with sleep begin? What was happening in your life at that time, or a few months before?
14. Are your sheets and blankets in extreme disarray in the morning when you wake up?
15. Do you awaken yourself by kicking your legs during the night? Has your bed partner ever complained about it?
16. Has your bed partner ever said that you are a heavy snorer, that you stopped breathing for more than ten seconds, or that you have trouble breathing?
17. Do you currently have nightmares or night terrors?
18. Do you grind or clench your teeth at night?
19. Have you often wet the bed as an adult?
20. Have you often walked in your sleep as an adult?

of sleep you get now. Keep the answers for future reference so that you can see your improvement after being on the program.

Looking over these questions now can give you some feeling for what might be causing your insomnia and suggest what parts of our program you may want to concentrate on. For example, questions 1 through 4 assess the regularity of your sleep-wake behavior. Most people's bedtime and waking times vary no more than about one hour from day to day. If yours vary more, that may be part of your problem, and you would learn how to deal with it in the sections of the program on setting up a regular sleep schedule.

If weeknights are much different from weekends, it may be that you are depriving yourself of sleep during the week. Can you give yourself more time to sleep? Some people lie in bed on weekends for hours after they have finished sleeping. That is not recommended for people with sleep problems, because it disturbs the sleep-wake rhythm.

Question 5: If you habitually take more than an hour to fall asleep, you may have excessive tension. Study particularly well the chapters on relaxation techniques (Chapter 7) and on managing stress (Chapter 8). Or, your internal sleep-wake rhythms may have slipped. In that case, study the chapter on resetting the sleep clock (Chapter 11).

Question 6: Surprisingly, most good sleepers awaken 5 to 15 times each night, but fall asleep within a few seconds and even may forget about having been awake. The problem is not waking up, but what happens then. If you don't fall back asleep right away, pay attention to the thoughts you have. They may give you a clue to your problem.

Question 7: Some people need more sleep, others less. This question, surprisingly, is relevant only if you are tired during the day (see questions 8 and 9).

Questions 8 and 9 are the crucial ones to help you answer the big question: Do you really have insomnia? Not everyone who thinks he or she has insomnia actually does. Not sleeping very much is not considered insomnia unless it impairs your daytime functioning or your physical or emotional well-being. As we discussed in Chapter 1, some people simply are short sleepers. They are lucky enough to need less sleep than most of the rest of us, sometimes only three to five hours. Since everyone else seems to need more sleep, they get worried that there might be something wrong with them—they don't sleep very long, so they must have insomnia. If you feel alert and energetic during the day, don't worry if you sleep less than anybody else in the family—it's okay. In fact, it's terrific—you'll have all that extra time to do the things you want to do.

However, don't try to be a short sleeper if you're not. You may be shortchanging yourself because of the demands of a job or because you are trying to prove you're a superwoman or man.

There also are people who have very poor perception of their sleep. They greatly overestimate how long it takes them to fall asleep or how many times they awaken during the night. Some people even *dream* that they are awake and only *imagine* that they have not slept. Some patients who believe they are getting only three or four hours of sleep a night are shown at the lab to be sleeping six, seven, or even eight hours.

If you are not sure whether or not you really have insomnia, focus on questions 8 and 9. Ask yourself this one major question: Do I often feel exhausted and unable to function properly during the day because of lack of sleep, possibly even falling asleep when I don't want to? If you answered yes, you probably really do have insomnia. If you are alert, are in reasonably good spirits, and are functioning well during the day, you probably are getting enough sleep, even though it might be only four hours or even two hours.

Other questions to ask to determine whether you're getting enough sleep: Do you have a very hard time getting up in the morning? Do you need an alarm clock to wake you up? Do you drop off to sleep in front of the television, when reading, or at concerts? Do you sleep much later than usual on the weekends? A "yes" to more than two of these questions would indicate that you're probably not getting enough sleep.

On the other hand, do you lie in bed for a long time after the lights are out wondering when you'll fall asleep? Or do you wake up in the morning hours before you want to get up? You may be getting more bed rest than you need—strangely enough, one of the big causes of insomnia.

You may want to do your own experiment about how much sleep you need. Figure out how much you sleep now. If you are not sleepy during the day and feel fine, try sleeping an hour less. Sleep the new pattern for a week or two and see how you feel. If you feel sleepy during the day, the new pattern probably isn't enough sleep and you should return to the previous amount.

On the other hand, if you are now falling asleep during boring lectures or when watching TV or driving, you could try staying in bed an hour or so longer for a week and see whether that improves your sleepiness.

(If sleeping much more than you do now for a week *still* does not cure your daytime sleepiness, it may be that some problem is disturbing your sleep at night, something that you probably are not aware of. We will talk about some of these things in later chapters.)

Keep adjusting the amount of time in bed up or down, but always try each amount for at least a week, since it takes awhile for your body to get adjusted.

Get to know your own body and learn your own sleep needs. Don't worry about how much sleep you are "supposed" to have, only about whether you get enough sleep to keep from being tired. Find the pattern that suits you physically and emotionally, then follow the pattern.

Question 10: Napping is controversial. It hurts sleep at night for some people, but not for others. Cut out the naps for a week and see if it helps you to sleep better at night.

Question 11:. Shift work is very tough on those who sleep poorly. We will have much advice on this in the chapter on shift work and jet lag (Chapter 12).

If you answered yes to question 12, it could mean that you are a short sleeper or are going to bed too early. Your early awakening also could be a consequence of depression. You can determine whether you are a short sleeper by going to bed one or two hours later in the evening for a few weeks and seeing if you wake up at a better hour. If the early morning awakenings are a consequence of depression, the next questionnaire (page 29) may help you determine this.

Question 13: The start of a sleep problem often is associated with some important event in a person's life. Even if the event was positive, it may be connected with your sleep problem. For example, if you got a promotion and assumed more responsibility, it may have made you happy, but it also may have put you under more stress.

If you answered yes to questions 14 and 15, you may have what sleep specialists call *periodic limb movements* during sleep, which often disturb people's sleep. If you answered yes to question 16, you may have a condition called *sleep apnea*. We will tell you more about these important problems in the chapters on medical causes (Chapter 13) and other sleep disorders (Chapter 15).

If you answered yes to any of questions 17 through 20, you have one of the conditions that sleep specialists call a *parasomnia* that is disturbing your sleep. All these problems can be helped, and we will talk about them in Chapter 15.

Psychological Tests

According to national statistics and our own experience, at least half of all insomnias are caused by psychological problems such as depression, anxiety, marital stress, or job stress. (It does *not* mean when we talk about a psychological problem that you are crazy or psychotic, which is very rare in insomniacs.)

We find, however, that the insomniac typically is the very last person to know that his or her problem is associated with psychological issues. Like most people, insomniacs typically do not want to think of themselves as having an emotional or psychological problem. Therefore, even though you do not think your problem is psychological, consider that the chances are at least 50–50 that you might belong in this category. At the clinic, we often find that everybody around the insomniac knew that psychological help was needed, though the insomniac was totally unaware of this.

The kind of insomnia you have often is related specifically to a certain kind of psychological problem. For example, waking up too early is common for people who are depressed, while difficulty in getting to sleep often is caused by anxiety.

The Depression and Anxiety Questionnaires may indicate that you have a psychological problem, even though you think it unlikely. It might make sense for you to seek professional help for further testing and counseling. Talk about your situation. Ask the counselor's opinion about whether the basis of your sleep problem might be psychological. Try to listen with an open mind. If what the mental health worker says makes sense to you, listen to his or her plans for treatment and give the treatment a fair chance to succeed.

Testing for Depression

We'll tackle first the toughest question: Are you depressed?

Complete the Depression Questionnaire on page 29. These questions are designed around the characteristics of people who have

Depression Questionnaire

1. Are you often melancholy or sad and can't snap out of it?
2. Are you pessimistic or discouraged about the future, feeling—maybe realistically—that the future is hopeless and that things will not improve?
3. Do you feel you are mostly a disappointment as a person (parent, husband, wife, child)? Are you disappointed in yourself?
4. Do you find you are dissatisfied and bored most of the time, just not getting satisfaction out of things the way you used to?
5. Do you feel bad or unworthy a good part of the time?
6. Do you blame yourself—maybe realistically—for most things that go wrong?
7. Do you have thoughts of harming or killing yourself, or do you think it would be better if you were dead?
8. Do you cry a lot?
9. Do you get annoyed or irritated more easily than you used to?
10. Have you lost most interest in other people, with little feeling for them?
11. Do you now have more difficulty making decisions without help than you used to?
12. Have you stopped taking care of your appearance?
13. Are your bad feelings affecting your work?
14. Do you wake up one or so hours earlier than usual and find it hard to get back to sleep?
15. Are you tired even when there is no reason?
16. Is your appetite poor? Or do you eat excessively?
17. Have you lost interest in sex?
18. Do you feel worse in the morning, better in the evening?
19. Do you now have trouble getting things accomplished that used to be easy to do, such as housework or tasks at work?
20. Have any of your close relatives ever been hospitalized for depression?

depression. If you answered yes to four or more questions, you should consider the possibility that you are suffering from depression. Six or more "yes" answers make it imperative that you seek professional help. Getting treatment for depression often can solve an insomnia problem.

When answering these questions, some insomniacs readily admit that they are depressed, but claim that it is all because of their insomnia: "If I could just sleep better, I would not be depressed." True, there often is a vicious circle. Poor sleep leads to a worsening of one's mood, which then leads to worse sleep and even further depression. But no matter what the underlying causes, depression needs to be treated, either in therapy or with antidepressant medications.

Sometimes, depression is well-disguised. There is a clinical situation called *smiling depression,* in which the patient denies feeling depressed—while laughing and smiling a lot. Insomnia is the only sign that things are not well.

One typical case was Ida Simpson, the 48-year-old wife of a local businessman, referred to the sleep disorders center for serious and chronic insomnia of 18 months' duration. Trials with different sleeping pills had been unsuccessful. Mrs. Simpson appeared for her interview weak from lack of sleep and with bloodshot eyes, but well in control of herself. She responded appropriately, with a polite, tired smile. She said that her sleep quality had fluctuated for years, but that during the past 18 months, it had deteriorated relentlessly. She could think of no reason for her insomnia.

A careful interview revealed that about two years earlier, a number of important life changes had occurred. Her youngest son had gone to college, and neighbors who had leaned on her for support had moved away. But Mrs. Simpson felt that these events would have helped, not harmed, her sleep, because she had always dreamed about the time when, freed from other duties, she could start a new career.

Mrs. Simpson was admitted for three nights in the sleep lab. She averaged about 35 awakenings per night in the lab and less than four hours of total sleep. Much of it was stage 1; there was no delta sleep, and other characteristics of the sleep pattern were typical of depression. For example, the first REM period occurred ten minutes after she fell asleep, which often is a sign of depression, just as early morning awakenings are.

Extended psychiatric interviews and psychological testing over the next two weeks finally demonstrated a serious but extremely well-

Anxiety Questionnaire

1. Do you often feel upset or tense, maybe without even knowing why?
2. Does your heart often race uncontrollably?
3. Are your hands often sweaty, clammy, or extremely cold?
4. Do you often have a lump in your throat?
5. Do you have difficulties slowing down or relaxing?
6. Do you often feel insecure or anxious?
7. Do you often feel ill at ease?
8. Do you often worry about things you've said that might have hurt somebody's feelings?
9. Do you often feel tired without any reason?
10. Do you tend to worry, even over things that you realize don't matter?
11. Are you presently worrying over a possible misfortune?
12. Do you often feel nervous, jittery, or high strung?
13. Are you apprehensive about the future, more than other people?

hidden depression. According to her previously unconscious appraisal of her life, now verbalized for the first time, she felt incompetent, felt no longer needed by anybody, and was only awaiting old age and death.

An antidepressant improved sleep almost immediately. Then, in psychotherapy, Mrs. Simpson explored reasons for her low self-esteem and ways of becoming useful again. Eventually, she became involved almost full time in a charity organization. In a few months, she was off all drugs, functioned well, and said she slept almost like she had in her 20s.

Testing for Anxiety

Next, complete the Anxiety Questionnaire above. This set of psychological questions is based on the characteristics of anxiety. If you answered yes to more than three of the questions, you should consider that you may have poor sleep secondary to excessive anxiety. If you answered yes to five or more of the questions, you probably are more anxious or tense than other people, and your next step should be to seek professional advice. You may need some counseling, or your tension may be a bad habit. In that case, you may need to work with somebody who is skilled in relaxation training.

Also, think again about when your insomnia started. In our experience, insomnia based on tension and anxiety often starts either during a period of stress or a few months thereafter. As best you can, determine the onset of your sleep problems, and then look into your life around that time or shortly before. If there were important life changes at that time, they are likely to be involved in what is causing your insomnia, as was the case with Mrs. Simpson.

Think also about the things you are concerned about, things that are currently stressing you. For example, are you in financial trouble? Are you in the midst of a move? Are you lonely? Did you lose your job or are you afraid you might? Do you feel rejected or unrespected by your family? Are you upset over losing a loved one or because you fear you soon will? Are you worried about your marriage? Are you worried about things on your job? Are you not getting along with a member of your family? Are you concerned about getting old or becoming sick?

Any of these problems could cause insomnia.

Medical Causes

Now we'll tackle possible medical causes for your insomnia. Complete the Medical Questionnaire on page 33. A "yes" to any one of these questions might be the key to your insomnia.

Chemical imbalances in your body, hormone upsets, and other medical problems can cause you to sleep poorly. Therefore, if you cannot sleep, a logical first step is to see your doctor for a thorough physical evaluation.

Infections, an allergy, arthritis, back pain or any pain, headache, indigestion, coughing—and many other medical conditions—can cause poor sleep. It is important for you to know if such things are causing your trouble and, if so, to have them treated. Insomnia can be the first sign of a major medical disorder such as a thyroid or kidney problem that needs to be treated, and there are even a few life-threatening disorders that first present themselves as insomnia, such as

---

Medical Questionnaire

1. Do you have an allergy, congested nose, or coughing that bothers you at night?
2. Do you have arthritis, back pain, or other pain that keeps you awake?
3. Do you have frequent indigestion from eating heavy meals or from hiatal hernia or other causes?
4. Do you have other medical problems that keep you awake at night?
5. Do you take medications containing caffeine, ephedrine, or amphetamine?

---

certain brain tumors. They are rare; nevertheless, you should be tested just to make sure that you are healthy, especially if you are worried about being sick or if you have other unexplained symptoms in addition to your insomnia.

Insomnia is a side effect of many medications. This is true, for example, with many bronchodilating drugs for asthma, with steroid preparations, or with medications containing caffeine. Talk to your doctor about any medications you are taking and whether they might cause insomnia, or read the package insert yourself to see if it lists insomnia under possible side effects.

Alcohol and drug addictions also can interfere seriously with sleep. In one large national study, drug and alcohol dependencies were named as the primary causes of insomnia in more than 12 percent of patients with chronic insomnia. If you use either alcohol or mood-altering drugs on a regular basis, you should consider that this might be contributing to your problem.

And sleeping pills themselves can cause problems. If you use them, answer the following questions:

- Do you take any medication to help you sleep more than once a week?
- If you are on sleeping pills, have they lost their beneficial effect, or have you had to increase the dosage to help you sleep?
- Have you ever worried that your physician might refuse to renew your prescription for sleeping pills?

Lifestyle Questionnaire

1. Are you under a great deal of stress at work or at home?
2. Do you smoke cigarettes?
3. Do you drink coffee, tea, or colas in the afternoon or evening?
4. Do you, on the average, drink more than two cocktails, beers, or wines per day?
5. Do you abuse any narcotics?
6. Do you exercise vigorously less than twice a week?
7. Do you often work more than ten hours a day or more than six days a week?
8. Are you always serious, never doing anything just for the fun of it?
9. Do you take less than two weeks of vacation a year?
10. Are any relationships with your family, friends, or co-workers unsatisfactory, or is there much stress in some important relationship?

- Have you ever stopped taking sleeping pills and found that you slept almost not at all the following night or two?

If you said yes to any of the above, you should benefit greatly when you read the chapter on sleeping pills (Chapter 14).

Lifestyle Causes

Perhaps aspects of your lifestyle factor in your insomnia. Complete the Lifestyle Questionnaire above. In the chapters that follow, we will help you investigate each of these factors in more detail, with suggestions on how you might improve that part of your life.

Sometimes, we design our lives in ways that don't fit our body's needs; this can cause insomnia. Humans need regular periods of work, play, and rest, and the lifestyle questions are designed to see if you are getting the right balance. There must be a rhythm to our lives, an ebb and flow. It seems we are like a motor that should not be run at steady peak capacity; otherwise, we will burn out. We know that there are some people who can break the cultural norms much more easily than others and work at full tilt every day for 18 hours (just as there are motors that can put out much more work than others). However, if you have insomnia, think about your work-rest schedule. Are you running beyond the limits that nature designed for you?

Andy Owens was a 32-year-old businessman who ran his motor fast. Having started with less than $200 when he was 18, he had now built up a business empire worth more than $10 million. He had done it by very hard and carefully planned work. As his empire grew, he became busier and busier. Soon, he worked 16 to 18 hours each day, including Saturdays and Sundays (although for Christmas and Easter, he knocked off at 5 P.M.).

After a while, his sleep began to deteriorate. He had frequent, long awakenings at night. Not one to waste time, he started working on his business affairs during these awakenings, too. However, he found that he then "lost steam" during the day after having worked all night. He started to take naps.

Over the next two years, Mr. Owens developed a pattern where he worked continuously for two or three hours, pushing himself to the limits of his endurance, then collapsed for a 30-to 60-minute nap. As soon as he awoke, he pushed himself again, through night and day, weekdays and weekends. Not surprisingly, his work quality suffered— but this simply meant to him that he had to push himself harder. He held out hope that his business affairs soon would be so well settled that they would run by themselves, and then he could relax. However, that day never came, and his work performance continued to deteriorate. He was aware of this and became seriously depressed. A suicide attempt finally brought him to a hospital, where he was forced to reexamine his lifestyle.

Rarely are our patients as extreme as Mr. Owens, but there often is a long and embarrassed silence when we ask insomniac patients what they do for fun or recreation or what they would do if they were forbidden to work for the week. How is it with you?

Your lifestyle can be one of the most important factors causing sleep problems—and it is correctable in most cases. We will deal with many lifestyle changes in the program.

Sally Carson was a typical example of insomnia caused by lifestyle. She came to see us after she was fired for falling asleep on her job frequently. She was a medical technician, spending most of her days looking into a microscope. She had had no problem with sleeping during her college training, but developed insomnia as soon as she started her first job. She had now stuck it out for six months on the job, sleeping worse and worse and becoming sleepier and sleepier during the day.

When we analyzed her situation, she realized that the onset of her insomnia just as she got her first job clearly indicated that something was wrong with the transition from student life to a full-time job. However, she liked her job, felt that her supervisor was very fair, and was pleased that she now was able to make her own money, rather than depending on her parents. She felt that there was absolutely no reason for her insomnia.

But looking further, Ms. Carson realized that after she started her job, she spent her life between work and watching TV at home. Although she was quite shy, dormitory life in college had provided plenty of opportunities to socialize and talk. Living in an apartment by herself and looking at a microscope all day meant that there was no built-in need to interact with other people. She did not know how to make contacts, and she felt desperately lonely without being aware of it.

There was no need to give her sleeping pills—it was her social life that needed treatment. She had to push herself, join some groups (even though this was hard for her at first), learn how to make friends, and fill her need for human interactions. Six months later, she was secretary in a young people's church group, was involved in a volunteers' group reading to the elderly, and had found a boyfriend— and hardly remembered that she ever had insomnia.

Often, insomniac patients are aware of the stresses that cause their poor sleep, but feel trapped. They may feel they have to work for an overly demanding boss for financial reasons, or that they have to stick it out in an unhappy marriage for the kids' sake. Occasionally, this is true and, after careful consideration, a patient might decide that insomnia is the lesser of the two evils. Just as often, however, insomniacs overlook some possibility to change the stressful situation.

For example, one patient, Rita Fry, realizing that her marriage was on the rocks, said she was never able to talk to her husband because he always claimed he was too busy or too tired or wanted to watch a game on TV. She was advised to try again. Marriage without talking isn't much. She got up her courage and told her husband that there was something extremely important the two had to discuss, that it would take at least three hours, and that he had to put the three hours into his appointment book sometime over the next month, no matter how tired or busy he was. In exchange, she promised not to nag him for more time during that month. He reluctantly agreed. She decided that they had to go away for the three hours and selected a secluded spot where they could talk uninterrupted.

Mrs. Fry told her husband, as honestly and unemotionally as she could, how unfulfilled and lonely she felt in their marriage. He first belittled what she said, but since he had agreed to a three-hour session and there was nothing else for him to do, he remained with her and finally admitted that he, too, was unhappy that their previous romance had gone stale. They made plans to remedy the situation by carefully blocking out some times, even entire weekends, when they would be with each other. It worked, and she started to sleep better after their second weekend away from home.

In this case, the direct approach helped. In other cases, a counselor may be needed, or there may be no solution. If so, it's better to know it.

In later chapters, we will help you investigate, with open eyes, whether something can be done about your stress. Do not give up the situation as hopeless—there could be ways to improve it.

Sleep Hygiene Analysis

Lastly, we'll investigate your sleep hygiene. Complete the Sleep Hygiene Questionnaire on page 38. A "yes" to any one of these questions means that you need to think about that area and investigate it further. We will give you details for dealing with sleep hygiene problems in Chapter 6.

If your bed has become a sexual battlefield and you lie awake frustrated and angry while your partner sleeps, you may have built up negative feelings because of the arguments or the frustration. Insomnia often reflects an interpersonal problem, and you may need to solve your interpersonal problem to cure your insomnia.

No matter what originally caused poor sleep, over the years of chronic struggles with sleep, most patients develop poor sleep habits. The worst two are trying too hard to sleep and being conditioned against your own bedroom.

Sleep Hygiene Questionnaire

1. Do you often have feelings of apprehension, anxiety, or dread when you're getting ready for bed?
2. Do you have arguments in bed?
3. Has your bed become a sexual battlefield or the symbol of an unsatisfactory sexual relationship?
4. Do you worry in bed?
5. Do you often have feelings of frustration when you can't sleep?
6. Do you often have depressing thoughts, or do tomorrow's worries or plans buzz through your mind when you want to go to sleep?
7. Do you often work in the evening right up to the time you go to bed?
8. Do you often find you are trying to force yourself to sleep?
9. Do you sleep poorly in your own bed, but better away from it?
10. Do you sleep well when it doesn't matter, such as on weekends, but sleep poorly when you "must" sleep well, such as when a heavy day at work looms?

After not sleeping for a number of nights, you can't help but become concerned. Dragging yourself from day to day after not getting enough sleep is no picnic. So you start to worry about sleep and, when the time comes, you go to bed intending to really sleep well. Just the opposite happens! The more you need sleep and the more you try hard to sleep, the less sleep will come. And so there are millions of Americans each night who do exactly the wrong thing: They lie in bed, desperate, doing their very best to sleep. But this trying to sleep is exactly the worst thing they could do. The harder you try, usually the less you are able to fall asleep. This is one of the key factors in insomnia.

As Dr. Tom Roth, director of the Henry Ford Hospital Sleep Disorders Center, once said: "The longer insomnia lasts, the weirder it gets."

To find out whether you might have developed this poor habit of trying too hard to sleep, ask yourself whether you ever fall asleep when you are trying to stay awake; for example, when you're listening to the news or reading, when you're in a boring lecture, or even while you're driving. If so, but you then remain awake as soon as you try to sleep, you may be one of those people who try too hard. We'll discuss what to do about this later.

The other bad sleep habit is associating the bedroom and all that is in it with anxiety. When you lie in bed at night not sleeping, you cannot help but become frustrated. All the stimuli around you—the darkness, the feel of your pillow, your spouse snoring—gradually become associated with this feeling of frustration. Pretty soon, you are so conditioned that just going to your bedroom automatically triggers the frustration and wide-eyed awakeness. As soon as you go to bed, your eyes pop open just because of past experience.

To find out whether bad conditioning is at the core of your problem, ask yourself where you sleep best: in your own bed, or away from it. Many people sleep better in the living room, on the floor, in a motel room, at somebody else's house, or outdoors—anywhere but in their own bedroom. (We know a patient who found that he slept best while camping. So he snuck out into the back yard every night and pitched a tent.) If you sleep best away from your own bedroom, conditioning may be your problem.

What Did You Find?

You may have found that your insomnia seems to be due to stress, tension, depression, or anxiety.

You may have found that there might be medical or physical causes of your insomnia: an illness, medication, twitching of your legs, or breathing problems.

You may have found that your insomnia is most likely due to your lifestyle.

Or you might have found that you have learned insomnia: During periods of stress, you worried about sleep; when the stress was gone, you continued to worry about sleep from habit.

In the next step of the program, you are going to check out whether what you think is the cause of your particular insomnia really is. Just like the patients who come to a sleep disorders center, you are going to learn the secrets of keeping a Sleep Log and a Day Log.

···· 3 ····

Keeping a Sleep Log

A scientist's unproven idea is called a hypothesis; hypotheses need to be tested to see if true. This is what you will do now that you have an idea of what might be causing your insomnia. You will test your hypothesis to see if it is right.

To do this, you will keep a Sleep Log (page 42), on which you record how well you sleep each night, and a Day Log (page 43), on which you record what you did and how you felt the day before. These logs will help you determine what factors cause you to sleep poorly and which treatments and changes most likely will help you sleep better. This detective work will last over many weeks.

Although keeping these logs may seem time-consuming, it's very important that you do it. We've found that these logs are the most efficient way to discover what's causing your own personal insomnia. You can't know how to fix your insomnia unless you first know what causes it.

Almost every patient who comes to any sleep disorders center keeps a Sleep Log. At the beginning, many patients object to keeping a log. They say that there are no fluctuations in their insomnia—each night is as bad as any other. But if you'll fill out the Sleep Log every day for a week, you'll find that every night is not exactly the same as every other.

Other patients claim that their insomnia comes out of the blue: "I can never predict when I am going to have a bad night, and I never know the reason afterward." Sleep researchers, however, know that most things have causes and effects—including sleepless nights.

It's up to you to figure out what causes *your* particular problem. You have some ideas from reading the previous chapter. Now, with the Sleep Log and the Day Log, you can test those ideas.

Setting Up the Sleep Log

The first log you are going to keep is your Sleep Log (page 42). Here's how to set it up. Take one piece of paper for each week (you can copy the one in this book or draw your own). Make seven headings across the top, one for each day of the week and its date. Then make eleven headings down the left side, one for each of the items shown on the Sleep Log.

You should fill out your Sleep Log every morning about 30 minutes after you get up. For the date, give the date when your night began, not the date of the morning. In other words, if you fill out the Sleep Log on the morning of April 7, give the date as April 6. Guess the times as best you can, and don't worry if they're not precisely right. You are interested in general feelings and trends—how you rate your night's sleep.

It is important to fill out the Sleep Log *each morning*. When you write down your impression of each night, give what you think is true for that morning and the night just passed, no matter how the other days and nights look. For example, although it might have taken you two hours to fall asleep last night, you might be feeling refreshed and restored in the morning. If that is true, write it down just as it happened.

After you have filled out your Sleep Log for a week, it is time to pick out the one or two best nights and the one or two worst nights for that week. To do this, think of all the variables: how long it took you to fall asleep, how long you slept, how refreshed you felt, etc. There is no exact formula by which to weigh these different variables— it comes down to how you feel about them. Some people are bothered more by the long time it takes them to fall asleep, others by how often they awaken. No matter how you do it, you should come up with one or two best and one or two worst nights per week. Obviously, these terms are relative. We understand that you might not have had any good nights. If so, take the least bad and call it the best. For example, if it takes you four hours to fall asleep each night, but on Friday evening it only took you three and a half hours, then Friday is the best night.

SLEEP LOG

Please fill out this Sleep Log every morning about 30 minutes after getting up. Guess the approximate times. Do not worry if your figures are not absolutely correct. We are interested in your opinion of how you slept. Date the night when it started, not when you fill it out (for example, if you filled the log out on Wednesday morning, Oct. 5, the date of the night is Tuesday, Oct. 4).

Name _____

	SUN.	MON.	TUES.	WED.	THURS.	FRI.	SAT.
DATE							
Did you take naps yesterday? If yes, give total length of sleep in minutes.							
Did you take any sleeping medication? Give time and amount.							
When did you turn out your lights, actually trying to sleep?							
How many minutes did it take you to fall asleep last night?							
How often did you awaken last night?							
How many minutes were you awake during last night? Do not count the time it took you to fall asleep initially.							
When did you wake up for the last time this morning?							
How many hours did you actually sleep last night?							
When did you get out of bed for the last time this morning?							
Compared with your own avg. over the last month, how well did you sleep last night? Choose one from the list below, left.							
Overall, how refreshing and restorative was your sleep? Choose one from the list below, right.							

1. Much worse than my average
2. Slightly worse than my average
3. Fairly typical for me
4. Slightly better than my average
5. Much better than my average

1. Not at all restorative—derived no benefit from my time in bed
2. Some slight restorative value
3. Restorative, but not adequately so
4. Relatively satisfactory
5. Very satisfactory—feel completely refreshed and ready for the day

Name _____

DAY LOG

Date				
Sunday				
Monday				
Tuesday				
Wednesday				
Thursday				
Friday				
Saturday				

Setting Up the Day Log

The second log for you to keep is your Day Log (page 43). The Day Log is simpler to set up, but more difficult to fill out. You will use the Day Log to test your hypothesis of what might be causing you to sleep poorly. Record the events of the day, your feelings, and the various factors that you are testing. We suggest that you investigate about four of these ideas at a time.

This time, make seven headings down the left side, one for each day of the week, and four headings across the top, for the four variables you are going to test. These variables should include the things that you think are most connected with your own personal insomnia: ideas you got after reading the last chapter, or maybe just hunches. Some examples of variables that patients evaluate are shown on the sample filled-out Day Log on page 47. Others might include: amount of caffeine, amount of alcohol, amount of smoking, time and type of evening meal, upsetting telephone calls, upsets at work, upsets with family members. You can look at emotional factors such as tension, anger, or anxiety, and also at physical factors such as the temperature of the room. Even if you have a crazy, far-out hunch, test it. Many times, your intuition and hunches are right.

Most of our patients are dumbfounded when we first ask them to come up with theories of what might cause them to sleep poorly. If they knew, they say, they would not have come for help. They ask us what to write down. But you—the patient—are the person who knows yourself best, and you are the one who ultimately has to provide the clues to what might cause your insomnia.

After some consternation, most patients can come up with some factors that might affect their sleep. For the few who can't, we ask them to put down four possible factors in other people's insomnia, "just to rule them out." It is just as important to know what does not affect your sleep as to know what does. Memory serves us poorly in this respect, though. We really do have to go about it in this scientific, painstaking way—noting down our observations carefully each day. We cannot just go by global memories such as "exercise never affected my sleep."

Whenever possible, we ask that you quantify (rate from 1 to 5) the variables you're investigating. This makes it easier to analyze your work later on. We do not worry about exact numbers. It is difficult to know whether your current mood, on a scale from 1 to 5 with 5 being happiest, might be a 4 or a 5. Simply do the best you can, trusting your own gut reaction.

It is important to fill out the Day Log before you go to bed, *before* you know how you will sleep that night. Then put it away until the next evening.

Evaluating Your Logs

After you have filled out the Sleep Log and the Day Log for an entire week, look at the two together. When you have identified the one or two best nights and the one or two worst nights, see whether any of the four daytime variables correlate with them.

Let's look at the logs on pages 46 and 47 as an example. These logs were filled out by Bertha Scott, a 30-year-old insomniac, who originally claimed, quite sincerely, that nothing at all was affecting her sleep and that her good and poor nights came strictly "out of the blue."

First, look at the Sleep Log. You will see that Tuesday night is clearly the worst, while Saturday and Monday nights were the best. What made Tuesday so poor and Monday and Saturday so good? Bertha decided to use a yellow highlighter pen to mark the good nights and the day's events preceding them, and a red pen for the poor nights and the preceding days.

At her conference at the sleep disorders center, she carefully went through each of the four variables charted on the Day Log. When she looked at "Exercise," she thought it possible that the intensive hiking in a state park all day on Saturday was associated with her sleeping so well that night. However, she also slept well on Monday night, after doing practically no exercise, and she slept poorly on Tuesday, after playing volleyball. It did not seem that exercise in itself determined her sleep, at least not from one night to the next.

Bertha felt that stress at work might be a factor, since she worked for a very moody supervisor. The good night (Monday) came after a day of some moodiness by the supervisor, while the poor night came after an average day. The other good night occurred on a Saturday when the mood of the supervisor could not be a factor. There was no clear trend in these data, so she decided to rate the mood of the supervisor for one more week.

Sample Sleep Log

Please fill out this Sleep Log every morning about 30 minutes after getting up. Guess the approximate times. Do not worry if your figures are not absolutely correct. We are interested in your opinion of how you slept. Date the night when it started, not when you fill it out (for example, if you filled the log out on Wednesday morning, Oct. 5, the date of the night is Tuesday, Oct. 4).

Name **Bertha Scott**

DATE	SUN. 10/2	MON. 10/3	TUES. 10/4	WED. 10/5	THURS. 10/6	FRI. 10/7	SAT. 10/8
Did you take naps yesterday? If yes, give total length of sleep in minutes.	No	No	No	No	No	No	No
Did you take any sleeping medication? Give time and amount.	No	No	No	No	No	No	No
When did you turn out your lights, actually trying to sleep?	11:00	11:00	11:30	10:30	11:00	12:30	11:00
How many minutes did it take you to fall asleep last night?	15	30	120	60	45	10	30
How often did you awaken last night?	3	1	4	2	2	2	1
How many minutes were you awake during last night? Do not count the time it took you to fall asleep initially.	45	15	60	30	30	45	10
When did you wake up for the last time this morning?	5:00	6:00	5:30	5:30	6:15	7:00	7:00
How many hours did you actually sleep last night?	5	6	3	5½	6	5½	7½
When did you get out of bed for the last time this morning?	6:30	6:30	6:30	6:30	6:30	7:15	8:00
Compared with your own avg. over the last month, how well did you sleep last night? Choose one from the list below, left.	3	4	1	2	3	3	4
Overall, how refreshing and restorative was your sleep? Choose one from the list below, right.	3	5	2	4	3	3	5

1. Much worse than my average
2. Slightly worse than my average
3. Fairly typical for me
4. Slightly better than my average
5. Much better than my average

1. Not at all restorative—derived no benefit from my time in bed
2. Some slight restorative value
3. Restorative, but not adequately so
4. Relatively satisfactory
5. Very satisfactory—feel completely refreshed and ready for the day

SAMPLE DAY LOG

Name **Bertha Scott**

Date	Amt. & Type of Exercise 10=Max	Mood of my Supervisor 1=Foul, 10=Happy	Telephone Calls in the Evening	Times I Felt Like Speaking Up, But Did Not
Sunday 10/2	Swimming, 10 laps 8	—	7:10 Jim called—we are apparently through 10:10 Rosie asks for recipe	Noon: Church meal, RE: pledge campaign
Monday 10/3	None 1	3 in a.m., up to 7 in p.m. (actually smiled!)	6:50 Joe RE: banquet 8:30 Doris (chat)	—
Tuesday 10/4	Volleyball 7	5 all day	8:50 My mother—upset at my breaking up with Jim	—
Wednesday 10/5	Swimming, 20 laps 9	1 and worse! Nothing was right!	8:30 Doris again 9:15 Joe RE: banquet	10:00 At work RE: my part affiliation 2:15 Boss unhappy about my "slowness"
Thursday 10/6	None 1	7 Tries to make up for yesterday	No calls	6:30 Dinner with Doris RE: coworker
Friday 10/7	None 1	10 (I do not know why)	7:50 Jim—still angry 10:00 Salesman for trip	5:30 Beautician RE: common friend
Saturday 10/8	Hiking in a state park all day 10	—	6:20 my sister RE: Jim 7:15 Doris	—

Another hypothesis was that telephone calls in the evening might be significant—and this idea turned out to be a breakthrough. She was looking at the logs when, suddenly, she became very emotional. She shook, shouted, swore, and cried. After she calmed down, she talked about Tuesday night.

She was very surprised that her mother's phone call apparently was connected to her poor sleep that night. In the past, Bertha and her mother had had terrible arguments. She had accused her mother of meddling in her affairs and had even used an unlisted phone number for awhile, to avoid her mother's calls. However, she felt that she and her mother now got along well and were friends. She knew that the Tuesday phone call had irritated her "a little," but felt that she had gotten over it quickly. Her very emotional reaction in the office and her poor sleep on Tuesday night convinced her that this was not true.

We suggested that Bertha might keep these logs for another few weeks to see whether any new telephone calls from her mother would cause similar poor sleep. Often, it is good to confirm a hunch before acting on it. However, after considerable discussion of the issues, Bertha felt that she knew enough and wanted to remedy the situation. She resolved to visit her mother the following weekend. This was not an easy trip. She knew that simply yelling at her mother would only reinforce the old patterns. So she decided to think of the trip as a fact-finding expedition to discover why her mother upset her so and why her mother was still meddling in her life.

As she said later, the weekend was tough. Her mother, a widow living alone in a small apartment about 100 miles away, at first was hostile and severely critical. But Bertha stuck with her game plan of trying to understand the cause of her mother's actions and not to judge them. She kept asking questions, genuinely interested in what her mother had to say. For awhile, this confused her mother, who had been expecting a severe attack as in the past. Over the weekend, the two women gradually started to listen to each other's issues and try to understand.

Bertha's mother was feeling lonely. She also thought that she had let her daugther down while raising her and felt responsible for her daughter's difficulties. Bertha gradually realized that her mother was not the harsh, cold judge she had remembered from earlier days, but a lonely, elderly, guilt-ridden woman who constantly felt attacked, first by her husband and now by her daughter. There were tears and much embracing and a resolution to spend more time together. Not surprisingly, Bertha's sleep started to improve.

Stories don't always end with the drama of a TV script, as this one did. More often, the insights are small and the progress is gradual. Sometimes, if it is a relationship problem, a one-time session of sitting down and talking does not make that much progress. Often, therapy might be needed to work things out. Even if no resolution with her mother had been possible, Bertha Scott would have been better off knowing what caused her insomnia rather than feeling helpless because her poor-sleep nights came out of the blue.

The process we have described can be used to evaluate any hunch about what might be causing your poor sleep, as long as whatever you record on the Day Log is different on different days. You cannot, for example, find out whether coffee causes your poor sleep if you drink the same amount of coffee each day as you are investigating it. There needs to be variability. You could drink coffee on three days, no coffee on the other four. Also, there are things that take longer than a few days to study. Maybe you need to write down how you sleep now, then do two weeks of intensive exercise, and then do a Sleep Log again to see whether things have improved.

Your Sleep Log and Day Log will tell you something else. They will tell you what does *not* affect your sleep. That's important, too— then you don't have to worry about those issues. We know several insomniacs who ate very bland diets, hoping that they would sleep better. Even though they had eaten the same diet for three years and still did not sleep better, they continued simply because they had been told the diet would work. Another insomniac was told that reading in bed was detrimental, so he lay in bed for five years not reading, but also not sleeping. Had he kept a Day Log and a Sleep Log and read for a few nights and not read for a few nights, he could have saved himself a lot of sleepless nights—and not missed reading in bed, which he loved.

The effects of some things are a little trickier to measure—such as relaxation training, psychotherapy, or marriage counseling. In those cases, progress is gradual, and things sometimes get worse before they get better. Get one or two weeks of Sleep Log data before you engage in these treatments. After the treatments are finished, keep your Sleep Log for another two weeks. Compare the two logs and evaluate whether the treatments helped.

We cannot overemphasize that this kind of data, *carefully kept in writing,* is crucial. We have seen many patients who claim that a certain treatment has not made any difference. Then, when we sit them down with their logs, we find that, although they still might not be champion sleepers, they now sleep two or three hours longer. The converse is also true. We have seen patients who swear that certain treatments work, even though the data from the Sleep Logs do not indicate that they are sleeping better.

This is, perhaps, the main message of this book. Become your own personal sleep therapist. Do your own experiments. Set up your own theories of what makes you sleep better or worse and then test them with Sleep Logs. If the variable you study is important, you may want to do the experiment a second or third time, just to be sure.

You're in Charge

Being involved in solving your own problem makes you feel, rightly, that you are in control. You are not helpless—you are doing something positive to solve the problem.

As you test your theories, you may find that the cause of your poor sleep is something simple—like taking long naps in the afternoon or evening that keep you from sleeping at night. You may find that you were worrying, emotionally keyed up about something in your life. Perhaps you'll find something simpler: the trucks on your street that come by at 4 A.M. or the chocolate candy (with caffeine) that you have gotten into the habit of eating in the evening. It may be more than one thing—it often is.

Once you have narrowed down the possibilities, you can design a plan to conquer your poor sleep. Study the various steps of the program in the following chapters. We suggest that you read through these chapters with a pencil handy, so that you can underline or take notes on the ideas that seem most appropriate to what you have learned about your own problem. Try first the parts of the program that seem most pertinent to you; later, you can try other steps in the program that you think might help you.

For some people, the answer—and the cure—will come quickly and easily. Other people will have to try many answers—sometimes testing theories with the Sleep Log and the Day Log for weeks until they find what works for them.

· The important thing is to keep an open mind and keep working at it, choosing the steps that seem best for you to get back to a good night's sleep.

··· 4 ···

Three Things Every Insomniac Should Do

Dorothy Parker was an insomniac. Once, after desperately trying everything she could think of, she said, "I might try busting myself smartly over the temple with the nightlight."

One European king was reputed to own several hundred beds and rotated among them. A patient we know once counted 5,865 sheep before giving up—exhausted, but wide awake.

There are three things you can do that are much easier and will give you more benefit. No matter what other factors might be causing your poor sleep, you can do these three things immediately and have an excellent chance of helping your sleep.

The three things: Reduce caffeine, limit alcohol, and eliminate smoking.

We know how difficult this can be, so we are not going to insist that everyone do it. Instead, we want you to investigate for yourself the effects of these three things on you.

Reduce Caffeine

Caffeine and similar stimulants can cause many more problems than most people realize, and too much caffeine may be a factor in your insomnia. Often, insomniacs are exceptionally sensitive to this stimulant, they may be unable to sleep after one cup of tea or a chocolate bar in the afternoon. One study showed that patients who had caffeine-induced wakefulness cleared caffeine more slowly from their bodies.

CAFFEINE CONTENT OF BEVERAGES AND FOODS

	Milligrams Caffeine	
Item	Average	Range
Coffee (5-oz. cup)		
Brewed, drip method	115	60–180
Brewed, percolator	80	40–170
Instant	65	30–120
Decaffeinated, brewed	3	2–5
Decaffeinated, instant	2	1–5
Tea (5-oz. cup)		
Brewed, major U.S. brands	40	20–90
Brewed, imported brands	60	25–110
Instant	30	25–50
Iced (12-oz. glass)	70	67–76
Cocoa beverage (5-oz. cup)	4	2–20
Chocolate milk beverage (8 oz.)	5	2–7
Milk chocolate (1 oz.)	6	1–15
Dark chocolate, semi-sweet (1 oz.)	20	5–35
Baker's chocolate (1 oz.)	26	26
Chocolate-flavored syrup (1 oz.)	4	4

Source: FDA, Food Additive Chemistry Evaluation Branch, based on evaluations of existing literature on caffeine levels.

The concentration of caffeine in their blood was higher at midnight—eight hours after afternoon coffee—than it was in other people. Sensitivity to caffeine can increase with age. Even if you have had coffee, tea, or cola drinks in late afternoon or in the evening in the past with no trouble, they can start contributing to poor sleep as you get older.

Consuming more than 300 mg of caffeine a day (three cups of coffee or cola, or several caffeine-containing pain tablets) is likely to affect sleep and create the danger of caffeine addiction. In some people, it takes *much* less—one cup of coffee at lunch or one cola in the afternoon.

The tables on pages 53, 54, and 55 will help you determine how much caffeine you might be getting in your diet. Note that the amount

CAFFEINE CONTENT OF SOFT DRINKS

Brand	Milligrams Caffeine (12-oz. serving)
Sugar-Free Mr. PIBB	58.8
Mountain Dew	54.0
Mello Yello	52.8
TAB	46.8
Coca-Cola	45.6
Diet Coke	45.6
Shasta Cola	44.4
Shasta Cherry Cola	44.4
Shasta Diet Cola	44.4
Mr. PIBB	40.8
Dr. Pepper	39.6
Sugar-Free Dr. Pepper	39.6
Big Red	38.4
Sugar-Free Big Red	38.4
Pepsi-Cola	38.4
Aspen	36.0
Diet Pepsi	36.0
Pepsi Light	36.0
RC Cola	36.0
Kick	31.2
Canada Dry Jamaica Cola	30.0
Canada Dry Diet Cola	1.2

Source: Institute of Food Technologists (IFT), April 1983, based on data from National Soft Drink Association, Washington, DC. IFT also reports that there are at least 68 flavors and varieties of soft drinks produced by 12 leading bottlers that have no caffeine.

of caffeine in coffee or tea depends on what method of brewing is used and how strong you make it.

Symptoms that can be caused by too much caffeine include shakiness, nervousness, irritability, palpitations of the heart, upsets in heart rhythms, low blood pressure, circulatory failure, nausea, vomiting, dizziness, stomach pain, diarrhea, frequent urination—and, of course, insomnia. Caffeine has been shown to cause people to take longer to get to sleep, to cause more awakenings, and to lower the quality of sleep, even in people who are not aware of it.

Caffeine Content of Drugs

Prescription Drugs	Caffeine, milligrams per tablet or capsule
Cafergot (migraine headaches)	100
Norgesic Forte (muscle relaxant)	60
Norgesic (muscle relaxant)	30
Fiorinal (tension headache)	40
Fioricet (headache pain relief)	40
Darvon compound (pain relief)	32
Soma Compound (pain relief, muscle relaxant)	32
Synalgos-DC (pain relief)	30
Synalgos-DC-A (pain relief)	30

Nonprescription Drugs

Weight-Control Aids	
Codexin	
Dex-A-Diet II	200
Dexatrim, Dexatrim Extra Strength	200
Dietac capsules	200
Maximum Strength Appedrine	100
Prolamine	140
Alertness Tablets	
Nodoz	100
Vivarin	200
Analgesic/Pain Relief	
Anacin, Maximum Strength Anacin	32
Excedrin	65
Midol	32
Vanquish	33
Diuretics	
Aqua-Ban	100
Maximum Strength Aqua-Ban Plus	200
Permathene H2 Off	200
Cold/Allergy Remedies	
Coryban-D capsules	30
Triaminicin tablets	30
Dristan Decongestant tablets and Dristan A-F Decongestant tablets	16
Duradyne-Forte	30

Source: FDA's National Center for Drugs and Biologics.

Bernadette Baker, a 52-year-old mother of three grown children, came into the Dartmouth clinic for insomnia. She had always been very civic-minded and capable, and after her last child had left for college five years earlier, she became a leader in many organizations. But now she was "too nervous and high-strung to sleep." She suspected that her insomnia was caused by overwork, but admitted that she had been even busier—but sleeping well—when all the children were at home.

Over the previous five years, Mrs. Baker had been hospitalized three times for "nervous exhaustion." Each hospitalization was highly successful; her insomnia usually vanished within a week and she "slept like a baby." Unfortunately, the cure never lasted. Then she had psychotherapy because of the possibility that her need to work so hard was covering up depression from the "empty-nest syndrome." After a year of counseling, though, the therapist was not so sure and referred her to the sleep disorders center.

During a routine sleep history, Mrs. Baker's answers suggested excessive tension and agitation, but an otherwise healthy woman. Then she was asked, "How many cups of coffee do you drink?" She answered vaguely: "A few—I don't know. I drink coffee a lot—it's the only thing they serve during all the committee meetings." Finally, she guessed about 8 to 10 cups per day. A week's Day Log, however, showed an intake of about 20 to 25 cups a day.

Withdrawn from coffee, Mrs. Baker first became tearful, depressed, headachy, and lethargic—the typical symptoms of caffeine withdrawal—just as she had been during the first days of her psychiatric hospitalizations. Two weeks after withdrawal, the insomnia and agitation were gone. Now, four years later, Mrs. Baker is busier than ever and sleeps well.

To find out the specific effect of caffeine on your sleep, try the following experiment. Eliminate caffeine from your diet for one week. Have no coffee, tea, cocoa, colas, other caffeine drinks, or caffeine medications, such as headache pills. If, after a caffeine-free week, you find that you're less nervous and tense and that you sleep better, caffeine may be something you should eliminate from your diet permanently.

This could be difficult at first, because you may be addicted to it. In fact, most people have a headache for the first day or two as a withdrawal symptom, and it is not rare for a person to get very sleepy, have no energy, and actually feel sick. Or you may be irritable, depressed, or tense. If you are seriously addicted to caffeine, as indicated by severe headaches and lethargy with sudden withdrawal, you may have to withdraw from it gradually to decrease any headache, jitteriness, or depression.

There are other clues to caffeine addiction—waking up in the middle of the night unless you've had a cup of coffee at bedtime or waking up with a headache on the mornings you sleep late. If you usually have several cups of coffee in the morning or during the day, your headache at these times may be due to caffeine withdrawal.

If you often need to get up to urinate in the night or have trouble with urgency in the daytime, you may find that eliminating caffeine also eliminates this problem. One urologist friend of ours said that of the patients coming to him with these urinary complaints, two out of three eliminated their symptoms simply by removing caffeine from their diets.

But if you really feel that you want some caffeine in your life (don't kid yourself, you don't *need* it), you can try gradually adding it back into your diet to check its effect. Perhaps small amounts won't make any difference. If you wish, try adding one cup or glass a day of caffeine-drink back into your diet and test its effect. A few days later, add another, to determine just how much caffeine you can tolerate without becoming tense and staying awake. But be careful that your caffeine addiction and insomnia don't start all over again. It is usual to feel very good (sometimes euphoric) at first from the stimulation of the caffeine, but a few days later, your insomnia may return.

Some helpful tricks to reduce caffeine intake: Throw out the first cup of tea from a tea bag and use the second, which will have less caffeine. For the times when you enjoy a hot drink most, drink decaffeinated coffee and tea. Don't forget to count the caffeine in soft drinks, headache and other medications, chocolate candy, chocolate desserts, and chocolate-flavored after-dinner drinks.

If you are pregnant or are breast-feeding your baby, be very careful of caffeine in your diet. Babies can have disrupted sleep and colic symptoms due to caffeine nerves—from their mothers drinking too much coffee. And the Food and Drug Administration (FDA) advises pregnant women to avoid caffeine-containing products as much as possible.

If your older child has sleep difficulties, remember that when a child drinks a can of cola, the caffeine intake is comparable to four cups of coffee for an adult. Dr. Walter Silver, of Maimonides Medical Center in New York, reported in the journal *Pediatrics* on a group of adolescents who had insomnia and fast heartbeat, both of which disappeared when cola drinks were withdrawn from their diets.

Limit Alcohol

Many doctors used to prescribe a cocktail or glass of wine before bedtime for insomnia, but this practice is no longer recommended. Still, many people use alcohol as a sleeping aid. In addition to the obvious danger of slipping into alcoholism from daily use, there are several reasons not to use alcohol to induce sleep.

While many people find that alcohol at bedtime helps them to relax and fall asleep easier, others find that after drinking alcohol they can't fall asleep at all. And in nearly everyone, even if they've had only one or two drinks, drinking alcohol late in the evening produces troubled and fragmented sleep. The person does not sleep soundly, but wakes up many times throughout the night. By morning, there invariably is *less* sleep than without alcohol.

A single cocktail or glass of wine at dinnertime or a liqueur afterward probably won't be in your bloodstream long enough to cause insomnia at bedtime, but a nightcap within two hours of bedtime probably will.

As with caffeine, you can test this on yourself. If it is your custom, for a week, have a drink or two before bedtime and write down how you sleep during the night and how you feel the next day. For the second week, do not have any alcohol in the evening and see how you sleep and how you feel the next day. Then make your decision.

If you've been having several drinks each night and find it difficult to stop all at once, you may want to withdraw gradually. Cut down to one drink per night for a few days, then to one very weak drink for a few days. Then eliminate the alcohol completely and have a glass of fruit juice with ice instead.

If you are going to use booze to help you snooze, you must know the dangers. One is that alcohol produces poor-quality sleep; another is the danger of slipping into alcohol dependency. Many alcoholics have said that they started drinking regularly to try to get to sleep at night.

In chronic alcoholics, sleep patterns are quite abnormal. Sleep usually is very disrupted, often with hundreds of awakenings in a night. In fact, chronic alcoholic patients show a "prematurely aged" sleep, characterized by many awakenings, little or no delta sleep, and decreased REM sleep. Sleep is fragmented and shallow, total time in bed often is increased, the sleep-wake rhythm is blurred, and patients may show excessive daytime sleepiness. This problem may last months, if not years, after ending all drinking.

Babies born to mothers who drink heavily during pregnancy are found to have abnormal sleep patterns after birth.

In some people, alcohol is known to trigger or aggravate sleep apnea (stopped-breathing episodes), sometimes only to the point of violent snoring and snorting, other times serious enough to be life-threatening, especially if a person has a history of lung or heart disease. Alcohol worsens the condition because it relaxes the muscles in the throat and suppresses the awakening mechanisms.

At the University of Florida in Gainesville, 20 men ranging in age from the 20s to the mid-60s were given four shots of vodka less than an hour before bedtime. Their sleep was monitored, and the episodes of sleep apnea were five times more frequent than for the same men when they had not consumed alcohol. "For those already suffering from cardiac and pulmonary disease, even moderate drinking before bedtime presents a risk," the Florida researchers say.

Some chronic alcohol users, as they withdraw from alcohol, for awhile may have much *more* insomnia, with frequent awakenings, nervousness at night, and sometimes nightmares. Often, such heavy users will resume drinking simply to protect themselves against this withdrawal insomnia, thus perpetuating a vicious circle.

Once a heavy alcohol user stops drinking, sleep can improve dramatically in as little as two weeks. Depending on the severity and length of the alcoholism, however, more time may be needed. Sometimes sleep recovers *very* slowly. Even two years after total abstinence, sleep still may not be quite as good as that of nondrinkers; in some cases, sleep never totally recovers. It is unclear whether such sleep disturbances reflect permanent and irreversible damage caused by alcohol or whether poor sleep always existed and alcohol was used initially to self-medicate the sleep problem. Give yourself plenty of time—even years—for this withdrawal insomnia to go away, and if you think it would help you through this period, get professional help.

The most important thing of all in relation to alcohol is this: *Don't mix alcohol and sleeping pills.* Don't forget this! The combination can lead to serious side effects, each one aggravating the other, and can even be fatal.

Bill Quince was a 48-year-old car dealer and a bachelor. He was a very sociable guy and loved to eat and drink. Although he never married, he usually had a girlfriend living with him. He was an optimist, and in 1980 he built a much larger car dealership than he could afford. Then a recession hit. Overextended, he went bankrupt within six months. His girlfriend left. Mr. Quince took to eating and drinking alone and gained 25 pounds during the two months after his bankruptcy.

His sleep deteriorated. He found himself waking frequently at night and was groggy in the morning. He thought that he was just having hangovers. When he continued to feel miserable and sleepy during the day, a physician felt that the problem might be insomnia associated with stress. He prescribed sleeping pills.

But Mr. Quince's sleep became *worse* on the sleeping pills. He now awoke more frequently and for longer periods of time. Taking a double dose of sleeping pills made matters even worse. He became so sleepy during the day that he could not even hold onto the job as a car salesman that he had found after he had lost his dealership. In addition, he started to develop heart problems and often felt his heart skip beats or race wildly.

It probably saved his life that his old girlfriend came to town, and they decided to spend a night together "for old time's sake." His girlfriend was shocked at what she saw: The man who just four years ago had slept soundly now could hardly sleep more than a minute without waking up, gasping and snorting for air. In addition, "he struggled and flopped around on the bed like a fish out of water." She got him to a sleep disorders center, where severe sleep apnea was diagnosed.

In this case, it appears that the initial insomnia may well have been associated with stress. However, Mr. Quince's weight gain made him vulnerable to sleep apneas. Alcohol then aggravated the apneas, so that he awakened frequently, gasping for air. Then he took the sleeping pills and, because all sleeping pills depress respiratory activity, the apneas became even worse when he added the sleeping pills. Finally, the combination of weight gain, alcohol consumption, and sleeping pills caused the apneas to become so chronic and severe that cardiac arrhythmias developed.

Treatment initially was directed toward the acute problem. First, his apnea was treated surgically. Then Mr. Quince began the long road back to health. We treated his alcoholism, then withdrew him from the sleeping pills. Finally, we had him increase exercise and lose weight. Now, four years later, he again sleeps soundly.

Getting Rid of Cigarettes

Often, where there's smoking, there's insomnia.

Nicotine can keep you awake. It's a stimulant, just as caffeine is. So if you light a cigarette when you are unable to sleep, you may want to change your behavior. Pick up a book instead—you'll have the added benefit of decreasing the hazard of fire, since you won't be smoking in bed as you try to fall asleep.

A number of studies have provided clear evidence that cigarette smoking causes sleep difficulties. Surveys show that insomnia ranks near the top of complaints expressed by smokers.

Smokers have greater difficulty falling asleep, because cigarettes raise blood pressure, speed up the heart rate, and stimulate brain-wave activity. Smokers also tend to wake up more in the middle of the night, possibly because their body is experiencing withdrawal symptoms.

Experiments by Dr. Anthony Kales and his team at Pennsylvania State University showed that when a group of men who had smoked from one to three packs of cigarettes a day for at least two years stopped smoking, they fell asleep faster and woke less during the night. Their improvement occurred despite daytime cigarette-withdrawal symptoms of temporary irritation, tension, fatigue, and restlessness.

So if you are a smoker, deciding to quit might very well help to cure your insomnia as well as help you live longer.

Test this for yourself if you wish, although it's logical to be a nonsmoker even if it has nothing to do with your poor sleep. When you have decided to quit, take extra vitamin and mineral supplements rich in B vitamins, vitamin C, calcium, and magnesium to help with the tension; stay away from smokers; and lay in a supply of fruit juice, chewing gum, carrots, celery, popcorn, and other snacks to help you through the first rough days. Then make the big move. Stop smoking for a month and see if your sleep improves.

Some people can quit with just these measures, but for many people, the rate of success is better with professional help. You may want to consult with your physician, a psychologist, or other therapist, or try a stop-smoking program or workshop recommended by your physician.

The first few days may make your sleep worse, since you could have nicotine-withdrawal symptoms. But don't make your decision about the sleep effects of not smoking until you have done it for at least a month. Use your Sleep Log and think very carefully about whether you are having better sleep without the cigarettes.

Most patients have excellent improvement in sleep when they become nonsmokers, and the improvement is even more dramatic when they also cut down on caffeine and alcohol. Of course, other health benefits are an extra bonus.

···· 5 ····

The Room You Sleep In

Marcel Proust was so bothered by noise that he lined his bedroom with cork. When he traveled, he always rented the rooms on either side of the one he occupied to protect himself against noisy neighbors.

Madam Chiang Kai-Shek, it is said, took her own sheets with her when she traveled—even to the White House.

We don't recommend that you become this fanatical, but having the right kind of sleeping environment can be an important step in sleeping fit instead of fitfully. How can you make your bedroom the best it can be for a good night's sleep?

Check the Simple Things

Are your sheets fresh? Is your blanket too light, too heavy, too scratchy, or too hot? Is your bedroom too hot or too cold? Are your pajamas or gown comfortable? Do you have a restless dog, cat, or bird scratching around in your bedroom at night?

These things could be interfering with your sleep more than you realize. Change them for a few nights, and see how you sleep then.

Check Your Bed

To make sure your bed is in good shape and not making you uncomfortable at night, check the following:

Is the mattress lumpy, does it sag on the edges or in the middle, or is it dusty? If these things are a problem, it may be time to buy a new mattress and box springs.

Perhaps your bed is not big enough, especially if there are two of you sleeping in it. Did you know that if two people sleep in a full-size double bed, each has only as much width as in a baby's crib? If you sleep with someone, try using a king- or queen-size bed, or put two twin beds side by side—you might sleep better. (A twin is 39 by 75 inches or extra long at 80 inches, a full double bed is 54 by 75 inches or extra long at 80 inches, a queen is 60 by 80 inches, a king is 76 by 80 inches, and a California king is 72 by 84 inches.)

Is your pillow comfortable? Maybe you need a new one. Get whatever you like: soft or firm, foam or goosedown.

Are your sheets comfortable? Satin sheets may be sexy, but they may be too slippery or nonbreathing for comfort. If muslin sheets are too rough, buy smooth cotton percale.

If you decide to buy a new mattress or bed, decide what basic mattress type you want: innerspring, foam, or waterbed.

If you decide on innerspring, check for the firmness most comfortable for you—the thicker the wire and the more turns, the firmer the support. Decide in the direction of too firm rather than too soft, since mattresses tend to get softer with age.

If you decide on foam, remember that the heavier the foam mattress, the higher the density and the firmer the support. You also can get a layer of soft foam around a core of firm foam to give you both support and a soft feel. A foam mattress can be used on a box spring or on a platform.

If you decide on a waterbed, get a "waveless" kind with built-in baffles and a liner and heater. You also can get waterbeds filled with a gel-like material.

And there are mattresses that combine types, such as a foam mattress on top of a waterbed.

Once you buy a mattress, remember to turn it over and turn it end for end occasionally, so that you will get even wear.

But remember to put this all in perspective. True, you need a comfortable bed, one that does not give you backaches or other problems. However, in many cultures, people sleep on a hard floor without problems. Others sleep in hammocks that sag in the middle. Around the time of Louis XIV of France, people slept almost sitting up (check the beds in Versailles).

If you have back trouble, you should sleep on a firm mattress. Dr. Arthur Michele, in his book *Orthotherapy*, recommends that people with low-back pain use a bed board of 3/4-inch plywood, cut to one inch less than the dimensions of the mattress. Place the plywood between the box spring and the mattress for better support. In some hotels, you can request a bed board to be placed into your bed.

If you wake up in the morning stiff from arthritis, you may want to try sleeping on a mattress pad of sheep's wool. A study reported in the *Medical Journal of Australia* found that a woolen underlay decreased movement in sleepers and improved the sleep of many people with arthritis.

If you tend to get a stiff neck, you may want to get a special contoured pillow, or try sleeping with a small, soft pillow to avoid unusual angles or stress on the neck during sleep. Also, don't sleep on your stomach with your head and neck twisted to one side.

If you have problems with heartburn or have breathing difficulties, you may sleep better if your head and upper trunk are elevated about six inches. Elevate the head of the bed or, if you sleep with someone, elevate one side with a wedge-shaped pillow.

Noisy or Quiet? Light or Dark?

Some people need absolute silence and darkness to sleep. You may be one of them, so try eliminating as much noise as possible by using carpeting, drapes, or other sound-conditioning and see if that helps you.

While an open window or a draft can cause problems for some people, others can't stand a closed-in room or air-conditioning. Especially if the house is tightly sealed against outside air, they feel that they are not getting enough oxygen. Try your window open and try it closed, and see which way is best for you.

One man who works at night and sleeps during the day had trouble sleeping because of noise and light. He solved his problem with black walls, heavy blinds on the windows, and black drapes; in addition, he wore earplugs. It helped a lot. Another patient wears a sleeping mask over her eyes.

Should you play a radio or not? Again, you must test it for yourself. The National Research Council of Canada says that the noise level of a radio, even when tuned very low, can disturb sleepers. But it probably depends on the person. It helps some people to let the radio play quietly all night long. When they wake up in the middle of the night, they listen for awhile and fall back to sleep more easily. If you like music to go to sleep by, try an automatic-shutoff radio or a soothing record or tape. ("Goldberg Variations" of quiet piano solos was reportedly written by Johann Sebastian Bach in response to a request by a prince to help him overcome insomnia.)

Some people are bothered even by the ticking of a clock. Others fall asleep faster with a monotonous noise.

It appears that most of us can adapt easily to any relatively steady noise. It's the occasional loud noises—an airplane flying over, a door being slammed down the hall, trucks running by occasionally—that we cannot adapt to. In fact, loud noises disturb sleep even in people who say they are not awakened by the noises and cannot remember them in the morning.

This was tested in a Los Angeles neighborhood located close to the airport. First, most people interviewed said they had become used to the airplanes and were no longer bothered by them. Then, the researchers went to their homes and did sleep recordings there, hooking up the recording electrodes to little transmitters and parking a receiving truck in people's driveways to read the brain waves. They found that even people who had lived in the noisy neighborhood for six years or longer and who claimed that they were totally habituated to the noise still awakened frequently when airplanes flew over. Indeed, measured over the entire night, people in the noisy neighborhood had about one hour less sleep than people in a quieter neighborhood.

If you have to sleep in such an environment, a noise screen is probably a good idea. Have a fan running, or an air conditioner. There also are machines that produce soothing noises, such as the sound of the surf or the gentle patter of rain. Or you can screen out noise with a white-noise machine that produces a soothing neutral sound without pattern or meaning. (To get home-made white noise, tune an FM radio between two stations.)

We can differentiate between sounds in our sleep, too, so what's causing a sound can be important. A soft sound that suggests mice gnawing in the bedroom wall might disturb sleep well beyond its actual noise level. We may wake up if the baby whimpers, but ignore much louder traffic noises we are used to.

Probably most important: People vary widely in their sensitivity to noise during sleep. In an early study at the University of Chicago, we found that some people awaken at a bare whisper of 15 decibels above background noise, and others don't awaken until a disco-level noise of over 100 decibels is reached. In addition, sensitivity to noise increases with age, and women are more sensitive to noise than men are.

Wake-up thresholds also depend on the stage of sleep. The threshold even may depend on dream content. If the sleeper somehow incorporates the noise into a dream, it may be easier to sleep through it.

The threshold also depends on the need for sleep; as the need for sleep decreases during the night, each stage of sleep becomes progressively lighter, and awakening becomes easier. If you've been deprived of sleep for several nights, it is more difficult to wake you.

The Clock

Many insomniacs have an illuminated digital clock staring at them all night. When they have difficulty falling asleep, they watch it anxiously. If they wake up in the middle of the night, their first glance is toward the clock. No matter what time it is, it's always the wrong time.

For most people, the bedroom should be a time-free environment. Once you've decided to go to bed, it's time to rest and sleep, no matter whether its 1 A.M. or 5 A.M. If you can't sleep, it's time for distraction and relaxation—reading, listening to music, or even watching TV.

Obviously, it is important that you get up at the right time each morning. Thus, an alarm clock should be somewhere in the bedroom, but for nervous clock-watchers, it should be where it can be heard, not seen. We advise setting the alarm and then putting the clock underneath the bed or into the top dresser drawer. Then relax until the alarm rings.

Like any other recommendation, this one has to be tried for a week or two before you'll know whether it is helpful. One patient became so obsessed with time once the alarm clock had been put under the bed that he started to estimate what time it was every minute or so. Obviously, a time-free environment was not what he needed.

For some people, on the other hand, the clock is reassuring. They may feel that they had been awake, but the clock shows that they have been asleep for several hours.

Check it out, and do what's best for you.

Other Environmental Factors

Your room could be harmful to your sleep in other ways, too. If you have an allergy, an open window could be bringing pollen into your room and causing breathing problems. Or an old pillow might be musty, causing you to sneeze, cough, or have itchy eyes. You might need to clean under the bed and wash drapes, blankets, and bedspread to get rid of accumulated dust.

Make sure the room isn't too hot or too cold. Despite old beliefs, there is no evidence that an excessively cold room makes you sleep any better. In fact, cold feet can keep you awake—wear socks if that's a problem. An ideal temperature for humans has not yet been determined. However, we do know that temperatures above 75 degrees Fahrenheit seem to disturb sleep; people awaken more and move more in their sleep, and both REM and delta sleep are decreased.

It's interesting that when they are in REM (dreaming) sleep, humans are *poikilothermic*; that is, they lose their usual ability to regulate their temperature by shivering or sweating. REM sleep stages occur more abundantly later at night, making it likely that extremes in temperatures are more bothersome at that time.

Also, make sure the humidity is right for you. If the air is too dry, your skin may feel dry, your throat scratchy, and your nose stuffed up. On the other hand, if it is too humid, you may feel sweaty and warm.

Some people don't sleep well because they feel unsafe. If you live alone and are worried about it, you might want to have safer door locks installed, as well as a smoke detector and an electric burglar-alarm system. You also might consider having an extension phone at your bedside table for emergencies.

Should you sleep with someone? We are reluctant to bring it up, but Dr. Larry Monroe, of Ohio State University, once did a study in which couples who were used to sleeping together were studied, some nights while sleeping together, some nights while sleeping in separate beds. When sleeping together, they dreamed more (more REM sleep) and had less of the deep delta sleep that is needed for body recovery. It appears that it takes at least ten minutes of undisturbed sleep before such delta sleep can develop—and if one partner moves during those ten minutes and disturbs the other, the clock apparently is set back to zero and the ten minutes have to start over again. So, while we don't want to interrupt the marital bliss of readers and certainly do not suggest that everyone sleep in separate beds, if you have trouble with poor sleep, you might want to consider some compromise such as twin mattresses on a king-size base or some other arrangement that may allow better rest.

Perhaps you simply want to read one evening or are tossing and turning and feel constrained and don't want to bother your partner. If so, go to another bed for the night (and explain the problem so that your spouse doesn't think it's the beginning of the end of your marriage.)

Sometimes what happens is that people go to bed at the same time when one of the partners really isn't sleepy and is just being polite. If you're a poor sleeper, don't do it. If you are one of the people who needs less sleep than others, it is guaranteed to turn you into an insomniac.

Again, as we say with everything in this insomnia program—you must check out your hunches for yourself. Different things work for different people.

···· 6 ····

Getting into the Right Frame of Mind

Corrine Barnes came into the sleep clinic stretched out in the back of a station wagon on a mattress. Lack of sleep had so weakened her, she said, that she could not have endured the 3-hour car ride sitting up. A sleep history revealed that she habitually spent 22 hours per day in bed, rising only for 2 hours in the evening "to keep my husband company over dinner." Her household was run by a maid.

Mrs. Barnes usually dozed on and off throughout the day and night, but she often received visitors by her bedside. She had even organized a women's group that met weekly in her large bedroom. She had been a relatively poor sleeper since infancy, and her current sleep habit had started about ten years before, after a serious kidney operation coupled with depression. She felt that she never quite recovered from the operation, although she had been pronounced medically healthy by at least two physicians.

She hated the night and everything related to sleep. She spent many hours each night trying to lie still (only to find that every muscle in her body wanted to twitch), working to keep her mind blank (only to find that her mind was racing from one subject to another), trying to breathe deeply (only to find that she became dizzy and lost control). She said she had tried "every recipe for sleeping published in any journal or book" that she could find, but nothing helped.

Mrs. Barnes had always felt inferior, even as a child, and had been quite overprotected by her mother ("You know, dear, you can't play outside, you'll catch pneumonia or be exhausted"). Lying in bed unable to sleep reinforced her feeling that she was inferior. She was afraid that not getting enough sleep was going to ruin her life, so she stayed home more and more.

Laboratory evaluation showed that Mrs. Barnes slept in fragments of one-half to two hours, spread throughout night and day, with a huge amount of stage 1 (the transition stage between waking and sleeping), but no deep delta sleep and very little REM sleep.

Mrs. Barnes stayed at a motel near the clinic for a month. With the help of a close friend, her time out of bed was gradually extended from 2 hours per day to 16 hours. She was taught relaxation skills and given sleep hygiene information, and she came in every day for extensive psychotherapy to build her self-esteem. Gradually, her sleep became normal, and although she never became a champion sleeper, she returned home satisfied. She now has slept quite acceptably for the last five years.

Mrs. Barnes is a classic example of the three biggest errors that insomniacs make:

"The longer I stay in bed, the more sleep I will catch and the better I will feel."

"If I can't fall asleep, I simply have to try harder until I can do it."

"There is nothing worse than insomnia. It will ruin tomorrow and wreck my life."

The truth is that the longer you stay in bed, the worse you will sleep; the worst thing you can do is to try hard to sleep; and whether you sleep or not probably won't make much difference in how you perform tomorrow.

Here are some things you can do that may seem strange at first, but will help you build the right attitudes and habits to sleep better.

Rule 1: Cut Down Your Sleep Time

Remember, there are large differences in how much sleep different people need. Some people need three or four hours and feel happy and healthy all day, others need eight or ten. Think back to your life before your insomnia developed. How long did you sleep when you slept well? Or think back even further. Were you an exceptionally long or short sleeper as a child? If you can't remember, it is likely that you were an average sleeper; that is, you needed about seven to eight hours of sleep each night.

What happens if you're a seven-hour sleeper and stay in bed for nine hours? Contrary to what you might expect, it probably would not cause you to have two hours of insomnia each night. Rather, after several weeks, the seven hours of sleep would get spread very thinly over all nine hours. There would be some problems falling asleep, plus many long awakenings through the night. Most importantly, sleep would become very shallow, with much stage 1 sleep and only a little deep delta sleep. It is as if a given amount of water were spread over a much larger surface, no longer covering it well. This shallow sleep is much less restorative, and you wake up more tired and weak than before.

Naturally, you think that you did not have enough sleep, and you extend your sleep time even further. This causes even more shallow sleep and more awakenings and makes you feel even less restored. And so it goes, in a vicious circle. The longer you give yourself to stay in bed, the shallower and less satisfying your sleep will be and the more you are in danger of becoming a serious insomniac.

One of the first things we tell patients in our program is to *cut down on time in bed*. It isn't easy. Your body, having become used to staying in bed for so many hours, probably will rebel when you make it stay up late and still get up at the usual time. In fact, your body may fight it for several weeks and may make you feel terrible for awhile. But even though your body may tell you it is sleep-deprived, stick to the schedule of sleeping only the number of hours you used to sleep before your insomnia and be consistent about it—no giving in. After a few weeks, perhaps less, your body will learn the new schedule and you will sleep more deeply and intensively in the time that has been allotted.

It usually is quite difficult to stay up for the new bedtime when your body says you're so sleep-deprived. You may be exhausted, every fiber in your body calling for sleep. You'll probably start falling asleep if you try to watch TV or read. It will help if you schedule more energetic activities to help you stay awake: doing laundry, cleaning out a cabinet, or arranging a late card game with friends. Active movement and social interaction both help get you through those late hours when you used to be lying in bed.

It also helps you stay awake if you vary your environment. First work at your desk, then move to the dining-room table, then into the kitchen. Work with music for awhile, then without. Walk around the room a bit; stretch. Do five minutes of exercise every hour or so. Wash your face, first with hot water, then with cold. Brush your teeth, comb your hair, perhaps change your clothes. Open a window for awhile and do some deep breathing in the cool night air.

It's still easier if you have a partner. Maybe you know someone else who has insomnia, and you can help each other with a buddy system. Discuss your plans together. Give each other a call every night or get together to keep each other company.

Pretty soon, the fewer hours of sleep will become easier. You'll know it was worth it when in two to four weeks you find yourself sleeping more soundly and waking up with more energy.

Dr. Arthur Spielman, from City College of New York, has a quicker but more drastic program. While our program has patients cut their time in bed to their previous normal sleep time of, say, six or seven hours, Dr. Spielman has his patients cut down time in bed to only three or four hours. They go to bed at about 2:30 in the morning and get up at 5:30 or 6:30. Every morning they call his answering service to report how many hours out of their time in bed they actually slept. How much they actually slept divided by how much time they spent in bed gives them their "sleep efficiency." (For example, if you were in bed four hours and slept three hours total, your sleep efficiency would be 75 percent.) After five days, if your sleep efficiency averages 90 percent or more, Dr. Spielman lets you go to bed 15 or 30 minutes earlier. Every time sleep efficiency reaches 90 percent, another 15 or 30 minutes is added to time in bed until, after a few weeks, you have a normal amount of time in bed and sleep soundly.

If you use Dr. Spielman's technique, no doubt you will often be on the verge of quitting. But remember that by the time you are tempted to give up, you probably have the worst nights behind you. It would be too bad to quit just before reaching the light at the end of the tunnel. It often helps to fill out some Sleep Logs as you go along so that you can measure your progress. Remember how long your insomnia has lasted—and compare that with the length of the treatment to get to normal sleep. Most people get better with the Spielman technique in three weeks or less.

We usually start patients with the easier go-back-to-the-hours-of-a-better-time technique, because Dr. Spielman's method is so difficult to carry through. It takes extreme willpower to remain out of bed until 2:30 A.M. when you haven't slept much for several nights.

If your insomnia is associated with depression, severe sleep curtailment also might help your depression. Doctors Pflug and Toelle, two German researchers, found that going without sleep for an entire night helped many depressed patients. Instead of feeling sleepy, they became energized. These researchers treat patients by first keeping them awake at night, then letting them sleep normally for two or three nights until their depression starts again, then keeping them awake another night, and so on. Some patients use this technique in the several weeks it takes before antidepressant medication starts to work; others are helped by the sleep deprivation alone.

Choose the technique for cutting down sleep time that you think will work best for you.

Rule 2: Never Try to Sleep

"If at first you don't succeed, try, try again" may work in many areas of life, but it doesn't work at all in sleep. The truth is that the harder you try to sleep, the more likely you are to remain awake. Sleep can come only if you don't force it.

Think about your own sleep. Do you fall asleep when watching TV or reading, when you want to stay awake, but then become wide awake when you finally decide to sleep? Do you find it hard or impossible to sleep at night, but then come close to falling asleep when the time arrives to get up in the morning? If you answered yes to either question, your problem probably is that you are trying too hard to sleep.

What can you do to keep from trying so hard? We've all heard of counting sheep. Not many of us are shepherds now, but it still is a good idea to think of something boring. The more you concentrate on a task that does not involve much muscular movement and is relatively boring, the more likely it is that sleep will sneak in by the back door. This is why we advise most patients who try too hard to sleep to engage in some distractions in bed: Read, watch TV, or listen to quiet music. The idea is to focus your mind away from trying to fall asleep, so sleep can occur naturally.

If you do read, use a light that is adequate, but don't blast yourself with bright light. You need to read something interesting enough that your mind won't wander off and start worrying about not sleeping. Try to stay awake as long as possible. Read until your eyes close involuntarily. Turn off the light and drop the book only when you cannot read any more. The harder you try to stay awake, the easier you will fall asleep. The harder you try to sleep, the longer you will stay awake.

Sleep, of course, is best, but being comfortable in your bed watching TV, listening to music, or reading gives you more rest than if you were to toss and turn, frustrated all night. So even if you read most of the night, you will be better off the day after.

If you find yourself wide awake ten minutes after you turn off your reading light, you did not read enough. Take out the book and read some more. Especially in the beginning, you may have to do this a number of times. Eventually, you will associate reading in bed with falling asleep.

Don't look at the time you read as lost; think of it as bonus time. Steve Allen, a man who sleeps more than average—usually 10 to 11 hours per night—says he yearns for some long, sleepless nights when he could read. "There is no way to determine what additional number of books I would have read or written, what additional problems solved, what additional melodies constructed, what additional adventures launched upon, had I enjoyed more wakeful hours." He says, by the way, that his biggest hit "This Could Be the Start of Something Big" came to him in a dream.

Some "experts" tell people to keep a blank mind. It almost never works! You can control your mind for awhile, but as you get close to falling asleep, you lose control and thoughts come back. Don't try to direct your thoughts. Controlling anything, including your thoughts, is guaranteed to chase sleep away. So let your thoughts wander.

But what if your thoughts get stuck on some unhappy or bothersome issue? First, don't fight it—let it be there and then let it drift off. However, if it sticks there for long, it often is helpful to turn on the light, write down this bothersome issue, and plan to solve it in the morning. In the same way, if you have a great idea or your brain keeps telling you not to forget to do something the next day, turn on the light and write it down so that your mind can let it go.

But don't forget this: No matter what you do during the night— whether it is reading, watching TV, or listening to music, do not let yourself oversleep the next morning. Get up at the same time that you usually do. Even if you read one night until 6 A.M., you must get up at your normal time, even if it is 6:30. Otherwise, your body will simply learn to read all night and then sleep all day.

Rule 3: Don't Be Afraid of Insomnia

Many insomniacs worry a great deal about their insomnia. They have a real fear of their sleep loss (psychologists call it *agrypniaphobia*).

It's 3:30 A.M., and you know it because you've been watching the clock tick the minutes away for most of the night. In the morning, you have to give one of the most important speeches in your career, and here you are spending these precious few hours wide awake. At first you're annoyed, then you start to panic: "I'm going to blow this speech because I'll be so exhausted I won't remember what to say!"

Well, hold it. Even if you don't sleep one single second all night, there probably will not be any noticeable deterioration in your speech unless you panic. The amount of adrenalin that will flow when you deliver the speech will easily overcome the lack of sleep for one night.

Most of us have been told throughout childhood that getting enough sleep is important. Without good sleep, it was implied, we could not function adequately the next day. Believing this, we really did find that we functioned miserably on the next day after poor sleep.

• • • ● ● • • •

When I was a young researcher, I tried to prove the importance of sleep by keeping volunteers awake all night and then measuring their reaction times, their ability to solve puzzles, and their ability to perform exercises. To my chagrin, I found almost no loss of mental or physical abilities after one night of no sleep. Since then, such experiments have been repeated dozens of times in other labs.

My second lesson came soon after. As a sleep researcher, I often had to stay up all night working in the laboratory. Occasionally, I had to give lectures after such sleepless nights. I felt that those lectures were atrocious! I thought I was humorless, could not find the right words, could not think fast, and delivered a very boring lecture. At other times, after having slept well, I felt that I did rather well. When the lecture series was over, I asked my students to guess which lectures had come after sleepless nights. They couldn't tell!

This is typical. The truth is that for most short tasks, one sleepless night simply does not make much difference. There is some loss of performance, but it is very small, hardly noticeable for everyday jobs. We feel that we are doing very poorly after a sleepless night, but to others it is hardly noticeable. Only in highly critical or dangerous jobs do we

*need to be concerned about any decline in performance after a sleepless
night.*

· · · ● ● ● · ·

Don't be afraid of insomnia! Don't get uptight if you're having trouble
sleeping. You will be able to function tomorrow, unbelievable as this
may seem to you in the middle of the night. Once you know that it
is not that important whether you sleep or not, you will stop trying
so hard, and it will be easier to fall asleep.

Another facet of the fear of insomnia is that many patients have
low self-esteem. They feel inferior and think that they are unable to
perform as well as everyone else. They hate to be unable to sleep at
night because this "proves" once again that they are so incompetent
that they can't even sleep as well as other people. Not so! Many of
our most famous personalities have had insomnia: Mark Twain (who
dealt with it with humor: "If you can't sleep, try lying on the end of
the bed, then you might drop off"); Sarah Bernhart (who said she
slept best when she slept in a coffin); and Lewis Carroll (author of
Alice in Wonderland, who was a mathematics professor and worked
mathematical puzzles to calm his mind when he couldn't sleep). Other
famous insomniacs include the Roman poet Horace (who coined the
phrase, "I cannot sleep a wink"); F. Scott Fitzgerald (who wrote, "In
a real dark night of the soul it is always three o'clock in the morning");
and other notables such as Proust, Kafka, Kipling, and Nietzsche.

So the attitude you want to develop is that sleep on any particular
night is not really that important.

Rule 4: Let Rituals Work for You

Most people go to bed using rituals, some being more elaborate than
others. People may watch the news, change into pajamas or gown,
brush their teeth, let the cat or dog out, and say their prayers. As they
do these things, they find that they become more relaxed and comfortable. Sinking into bed and closing their eyes is just the last part
of the night's ritual on the way to a good sleep.

Animals do it, too. When dogs go to sleep, they sniff around for
a likely spot and circle it a few times, stepping down on the vegetation
to make sure there are no surprises. Then they curl up and go to sleep.

For insomniacs, it often is just the opposite. Because their rituals have led so many times to frustration and arousal, they become tenser as they carry them out. They may be okay until they watch the news, then they start worrying about sleep. Going to the bathroom and brushing their teeth bring on tension and fear, and they hate going to the bedroom and lying down because they expect, from long experience, that this will result in another night of frustration and failure. Many an insomniac has confessed, "I hate going to bed."

So, if a ritual does help, keep it up, whether it is reasonable or not. Charles Dickens moved his beds, wherever he slept, so that his head pointed north and his feet south because he thought it would allow the earth's electromagnetic currents to flow correctly through his body. It doesn't matter whether he was scientifically correct or not. A good night's sleep is certainly worth turning the bed around for.

On the other hand, if your ritual does not help, try changing it. You might brush your teeth immediately after supper, say your prayers in the morning, or sleep on the couch for a few nights if you hate going to bed. Play around with different rituals for the fun of it and to let yourself be relaxed.

A hard ritual to break is the sleeping-pill habit. If you have taken a sleeping pill every night for years, and you don't anymore, there is an empty spot in your ritual, a habit that is not being carried out. Anytime a habit is thwarted, people tend to get tense. (Just ask people who habitually read the newspaper each Sunday morning. They usually get very irritated if one Sunday it does not arrive.) It is no good to simply discontinue the ritual of taking a sleeping pill. Put something else in its place. Maybe you can have a glass of milk, or cheese and crackers, or do some deep breathing.

It's important to let children have rituals, too. Let them say good-night to each fuzzy animal friend if they want to, and allow time to read them a book, say prayers, and have a good hug. (And speaking of prayers, we recommend that you *not* use the one about "If I should die before I wake"—it's enough to scare anybody.) Try to avoid battles of will at bedtime (but don't allow them to get out of control) and see that getting into bed is a relaxed and peaceful time.

Remember that some children, just like some adults, are short sleepers. If your child isn't ready to go to sleep, it's okay to be relaxed about allowing him or her extra time to look at books alone. Many children are more relaxed with their door left open, so they don't feel removed from the rest of the family. And if they are nervous about the dark, it's okay to leave on a night-light. The important thing is to keep it a happy time.

Rule 5: Give Yourself Time to Wind Down

The brain is not a switch. If you are an insomniac, you cannot expect to work at full speed until 11 P.M. and fall asleep at 11:15. You need to wind down slowly. Take time to play with a hobby, read a novel, watch some TV, or talk to your spouse or kids. Don't wrestle with a problem or get into an argument just before going to bed.

There are many ways to wind down. Actor Burt Reynolds says, "I am a great believer in a hot bath, and hot tubs are the most underrated things in the world."

A study by Dr. David Bunnell of the Institute for Environmental Stress at the University of California-Santa Barbara backs this up. He found that when people sat in a hot tub in the evening, it definitely helped them to fall asleep faster at night. However, there was little effect on sleep when it was done in the morning or early afternoon.

The temperature should be very hot—102 degrees to 106 degrees Fahrenheit—and you should stay in 20 to 30 minutes. Some people then like to go to sleep right away; others find it best to wait one to two hours or more before going to bed. Some people, especially the elderly, get dizzy from this much heat. If this happens to you, or if you have low blood pressure, check with your doctor.

Another excellent way to wind down and get yourself into the proper frame of mind for sleep is a massage administered by the loving hands of someone who cares about you. There also are valuable massage techniques that you can apply to yourself. A do-it-yourself facial massage is soothing. Close your eyes, put both hands lightly over your face and, with your middle fingers, stroke your forehead in a steady, slow, circular motion. Slide your hands downward and make light circles around your eyes, then repeat the circular motion over your temples, then along your cheekbones and chinline, and finally massage the back of your neck.

· · · **●** · ·

When it comes to winding down, what is one person's help may be an-

other's poison. For example, I used to advise almost anybody who had sleep problems to go for a leisurely stroll around the neighborhood in the evening, "to stop and smell the roses" and chat with a friend here and there. This helped many people to fall asleep better. But then one patient said, "That was the worst thing you ever told me to try! I couldn't sleep all night after I went walking!" When we talked about it, I found that as he was walking leisurely, his mind started to worry about many little things, such as "What did the boss mean when he said 'good morning' in that grumpy tone this morning?" After some trial and error and the evaluation of some alternatives by using a Sleep Log, he decided that he could unwind best when he went into his cellar where he had a metal lathe. There he would work for an hour or two with tolerances within a few thousandths of a millimeter. While such work would drive many people wild, for him that was what he needed to clear his mind.

· · · **●** **●** · ·

What about sex? Should doctors prescribe sex for insomniacs?

Making love has been used for centuries as a way to get to sleep. In most people, orgasm results in deep physical relaxation.

Dr. Ismet Karacan and his colleagues, then at the University of Florida, decided to study the effects of sex on sleep scientifically. They asked a group of young adults to abstain from sex for seven to ten days while their sleep patterns were measured. Afterward, they were asked to come to the sleep lab within a few hours after having had satisfying sexual intercourse. The night after sex, most subjects reported that they enjoyed more relaxed and restful sleep, according to Dr. Karacan. However, in the polygraph sleep measurements, no difference was seen between that night and the others. "This illustrates the point," said Karacan, "that the EEG does not necessarily provide a total measure of sleep."

In our experience with patients, whether sex is a good sleeping pill depends to a large extent on how it makes you feel. If you feel at peace, cared for, and loving after intercourse, it might well help you sleep. But if sex is a performance task, is used to prove that you are still attractive, or if you worry that you might not have satisfied your partner or have been rejected by him or her, then sex could be the prelude to a very poor night's sleep.

Rule 6: Keep a Regular Schedule

Charles Ping, a 32-year-old golf pro, felt that his inability to sleep had ruined his career. As part of the usual assessment procedures in our lab, he was given a Sleep Log and asked to note each day for a week the amount of time he spent relaxing in the evening, the time he went to bed, the number of times he awakened, when he got up, etc. Mr. Ping's log showed extreme fluctuations. Occasionally, he was so tired that he would go to bed at 6 or 7 P.M.; other times in the same week, he would stay up until 2 or 3 A.M. at a party. Sometimes he slept late in the morning; at other times, he got up to give an early morning golf lesson, sometimes with only a few hours of sleep after a night of partying. When questioned, Mr. Ping claimed that this had not been a typical week, so we repeated the Sleep Log the next week. It soon became obvious that every week was "not typical." However, while trying to produce a more "typical" week for us so that we could assess his insomnia, he gradually started to move toward a more regular lifestyle, getting to bed and getting up at fairly regular times. With these changes, his sleep normalized even before the assessment phase was finished, and no further treatment was necessary.

There is no question that we are creatures of habit and that regular times to work, to relax, and to sleep are conducive to sleeping soundly. Our bodies work best at a regular rhythm. While there are people who can live highly exciting and irregular lives, if you have difficulties sleeping, an irregular jet-set lifestyle is not for you.

On the other hand, we have seen people so concerned with their insomnia that they have become rigidly frozen into a set of boring routines. They hardly dare go watch a movie or break their schedule to read an interesting book or get involved in some project for fear that it might hurt their sleep. If this rigid approach to life describes you, allow yourself to loosen up and be more flexible. You might sleep poorly after an exciting event, but in the long run, living a boring, rigid life may be every bit as bad for your sleep as excessive excitement.

If you are wide awake on a certain night, say because you have received exciting news, there is no virtue in going to bed at your usual time and staying there tossing and turning. Stay up and wait until you are really sleepy. Being a creature of habit is useful to a certain point, but it's not good to be a robot tied to the clock.

A similar issue concerns retirement. Too many people retire and then lead formless lives lacking in goals and mental activity. With nothing much to do, they watch TV much of the day and eat at exact times and always with the same people. Life becomes boring, and they often escape by going to bed early and sleeping late. Insomnia is sure to follow. Instead, get involved in something important to you, live a varied life, and occasionally have an exciting late evening—it will be good for you. Fill your days with physical and mental activity, and chances are that your nights will be filled with better sleep.

What about napping? Many books tell you never to nap during the day because it might take away from your night's sleep. This is not necessarily true. Many patients sleep poorly at night when they have an afternoon nap, but some patients sleep quite a bit better. There doesn't seem to be any logic to it. It might be that nappers are less desperate to sleep at night if they have already had some sleep in the afternoon. Being less urgently in need of sleep, they worry less and fall asleep more easily. Whatever the reason, be your own sleep therapist and do what's best for you, no matter what others say.

Unconscious Attitudes You May Have Learned

If you have suffered from insomnia for a long time, you may have adopted certain attitudes and habitual behaviors about sleep without even realizing it. These hidden attitudes and habits can perpetuate the problem.

For example, there is what psychologists call *secondary gain*. It sounds almost unbelievable that something as miserable and destructive as chronic insomnia could be associated with some gain, but such is the case. There are ways to use insomnia to advantage. For example, people are more willing to forgive bad temper, errors in judgment, or lapses of attention if you tell them you haven't slept well for weeks. You don't have to accept responsibility for your own problems if you can ascribe them, consciously or unconsciously, to your insomnia. You also can use it as an excuse not to do something: "I could get more done if I didn't have insomnia."

Sometimes, people use their insomnia almost as a badge of honor. Dr. Julius Segal, sleep expert at the National Institute of Mental Health, wrote in *Internal Medicine News,* "Many among us regard their inadequate sleep with a touch of triumph. Those are persons for whom sleeplessness has become something of a status symbol. If you are sincere and worry about life the way you are supposed to, they would argue, then you must naturally suffer from insomnia. It is a badge of success: like ulcers or coronaries."

Indeed, some of our clinic patients have argued that it is a sign of callousness to sleep soundly in a world as miserable as ours.

Some people even take pride in their insomnia, just as some people like to talk about their operations. It sets you apart and gets you sympathy at the bridge table or poker party if you can complain that you didn't sleep a wink last night.

And some people even make a contest out of who slept worst. Ogden Nash captured this hidden attitude well in one of his marvelous verses:

> He unwinds himself from the bedclothes each morn and
> piteously proclaims that he didn't sleep a wink, and she
> gives him a glance savage and murderous
> And replies that it was she who didn't close an eye until
> the cockcrow because of his swinish slumber as
> evidenced by his snores continuous and stertorous,
> And his indignation is unconcealed,
> He says she must have dreamed that one up during her
> night-long repose, which he was fully conscious of
> because for eight solid hours he had listened to her
> breathing not quite so gentle as a zephyr on a flowery
> field.
> The fact is that she did awaken twice for brief intervals and
> he was indeed asleep and snoring, and he did awaken
> similarly and she was indeed unconscious and breathing
> miscellaneously,
> But they were never both awake simultaneously.
> Oh, sleep is a blessed thing, but not to those wakeful ones
> who watch their mates luxuriating in it when they feel
> that their own is sorely in arrears.
> I am certain that the first words of the Sleeping Beauty to
> her prince were, "You *would* have to kiss me just when
> I had dropped off after tossing and turning for a
> hundred years."
> (Ogden Nash, *The Stilly Night: A Soporific Reflection*)

Conditioned Insomnia

Sometimes, when patients can't sleep for a few weeks or months because of some serious stress or disease, a kind of unconscious learn-

ing sets in. Without being aware of it, they gradually start to associate
the bedroom with frustration and arousal rather than with sleep. If
that happens, just going into the bedroom, turning off the light, and
lying down brings back all the old frustrations. Sleep evaporates. Many
a patient has said, "I can be dozing in the living room all evening,
but as soon as I go into the bedroom, I am wide awake." We call this
conditioned insomnia.

To find out whether this association of bedroom with arousal might
be a problem in your case, ask yourself where you sleep best—in your
bedroom or somewhere else? If you sleep best in the living room, in
the den, or on vacation away from home, but sleep poorly in your
own bed, you could be suffering from conditioned insomnia.

A college student once came to the clinic who showed a surprising
degree of this conditioned learning. He slept very poorly in his dormitory. When asked when he last had slept soundly, he was quite
embarrassed: "You won't believe this. I am a mountain climber and
about three months ago we were climbing in the Rockies. We were
delayed, had bad weather, and finally, darkness overtook us. We had
to spend the night on a ledge that was narrower than my bunk, halfway
up a steep precipice. Each of us hammered in a few pitons, and we
tied ourselves to the rock. My friends were deathly afraid and didn't
close an eye. During all my college days, I never slept so well! It wasn't
that I was tired. I have often climbed for a day and then was unable
to sleep in my tent. I don't know what happened, but hanging on
that ledge I slept like a log."

What happened was that the student was in a situation that was
extremely different from his bedroom. All the conditioned learning
that he had accumulated did not apply.

We see this phenomenon often in the sleep lab. Some patients
have serious insomnia at home, but then sleep soundly in the lab and
are quite embarrassed the next morning because they have slept very
well. Actually, it's quite logical: Sleeping in the lab with all those wires
attached is very different from sleeping at home, so the conditioned
learning does not apply.

The Bootzin Technique

An effective treatment for conditioned insomnia was developed by Dr.
Richard Bootzin about 15 years ago when he was at Northwestern

University in Chicago. His technique is a type of *stimulus-control therapy* and is designed to counteract conditioned insomnia.

Here are the steps of the Bootzin technique:

1. Go to bed only when you are sleepy.
2. Use the bed only for sleeping; do not read, watch TV, or eat in bed.
3. If you're unable to sleep, get up and move to another room. Stay up until you are really sleepy, then return to bed. If sleep still does not come easily, get out of bed again. The goal is to associate the bed not with frustration and sleeplessness, but with falling asleep easily and quickly.
4. Repeat step 3 as often as necessary throughout the night.
5. Set the alarm and get up at the same time every morning, regardless of how much or how little you slept during the night. This helps the body to acquire a constant sleep-wake rhythm.
6. Do not nap during the day.

During the first night, patients usually have to get up five to ten times and may not get much sleep. As sleep deprivation increases over the next several nights, it becomes easier for them to fall asleep. Soon, normal sleep is achieved.

Georgia Sawyer had been a somewhat poor sleeper all her life. However, four years earlier, when her 19-year-old son became involved in drug dealing, Mrs. Sawyer was distraught and reported that she was "almost totally sleepless for at least two months." She felt that she never recovered from that shock and reported extremely poor sleep on a Sleep Log filled out before she entered the sleep disorders center.

To everyone's surprise, especially Mrs. Sawyer's, on the first night in the lab she fell asleep within five minutes of lights-out and slept soundly throughout the night. There was an excess of delta (deep) sleep, as if she had been sleep-deprived. In the morning, she was embarrassed by her good sleep and claimed that she had not slept that well in more than a year. Sleep on nights two and three was poor by our standards (less than 80 percent of time in bed spent actually sleeping), but Mrs. Sawyer rated both nights as "much better than my average night."

Mrs. Sawyer was treated with Bootzin's stimulus-control therapy. It was a rough three weeks! The first night, she had to get up six times; the second night, eight times. The third night, she fell asleep after the second time up and thought she was cured. But hard times still lay ahead. The fourth night, she had to get up eight times; the fifth night, six times; the sixth night, ten times; and the seventh night, five times. For the next few nights, she needed to get up only once or twice. On the eleventh night, she fell asleep right away, for the first time in many years. For a few weeks more, she sometimes had to get up at night occasionally. But from the fifth week of treatment on, she never had to get up again and fell asleep within three to five minutes.

Nine months later, Mrs. Sawyer said that her sleep was good again. Although she still suffered a few poor nights each month, she took them in stride, using the Bootzin technique. Anxiety and agitation were no longer chronic problems, but developed only when she was under severe stress.

Not all patients have as hard a time as Mrs. Sawyer did. Typically, they are over the worst of it and sleeping much better in about two weeks.

By now, there are 28 studies comparing the Bootzin technique with other forms of behavioral insomnia treatment. In all 28 studies, the Bootzin technique was either better than, or at least as good as, the other techniques. If you think you might have conditioned insomnia, you have a good chance of getting over it using this technique. However, it takes willpower. And it takes some time to change your feelings about your bed and your bedroom. Some people can do it on their own, but most patients need a behavioral therapist to help them through the worst of it.

Note that Bootzin forbids his patients to read in bed or watch TV, yet reading or watching TV in bed was encouraged in our discussion on not trying too hard to sleep. It depends on what the problem is. If you are trying too hard to sleep and need some distraction, it is good to read or watch TV. However, if you have conditioned insomnia, the Bootzin technique makes more sense.

The Right Habits for Sleeping Fit

Here is a summary of recommendations to help you develop sleep promoting habits. Unwind before you go to bed, go to bed only when you are sleepy, and do not stay in bed longer than you need to sleep. Never try to sleep, for it will guarantee that you remain awake. Take sleepless nights in stride; you can function quite adequately after them.

Keep your sleep schedule as regular as possible. Beware of hidden attitudes like secondary gain and conditioned insomnia. Attitudes and habits make such a big difference in sleep.

If you build these habits, you can enjoy a quiet evening until that sleepy feeling hits you. Then you can stretch, yawn, and head for your warm, safe, comfortable, bed. Crawl in, snuggle down, and drift away to the pleasant dreams you deserve.

Bedtime Relaxation Techniques

· · · · · · ·

About ten years ago, my doctor said, "Hauri, go home and relax. Your blood pressure is high, and if you don't relax you are going to have some problems." I asked him how long I should relax. "Sit in a chair and relax for half an hour each day," he said. So I sat there in my easy chair and said to myself, "Hauri, you gotta relax, you gotta relax! You sure don't want any problems!" I sat there and breathed deeply. I relaxed, hard, for what seemed like a long time. Then I looked at my watch, and only half a minute had gone by! I thought I'd better relax more intensively. After ten minutes, I was a nervous wreck.

· · · · · · ·

Some people can relax easily; others can't. Those who have problems must be told more than, "Go home and relax." Physical and mental relaxation are skills that must be learned. It takes time and effort to master them. But once they are learned and practiced, they can have lasting effects on disturbed sleep.

Some insomniacs benefit from relaxation techniques, while others don't. If you are tense, learning relaxation techniques can help you. But some insomniacs are *not* tense, and they do not need relaxation skills as part of their sleep-improvement program. If you are truly laid back and relaxed, you might be one who does not need relaxation training.

In this chapter, we are going to explain specific relaxation techniques you can use for better sleep.

Tension

There are three main types of tension: psychological tension, muscular tension, and sympathetic arousal.

Psychological tension is characterized by anxiety and worry. Many thoughts buzz around in your head and you may feel keyed up, jumpy, or agitated. If you scored high on the Anxiety Questionnaire (page 31), you probably have high psychological tension.

Muscular tension shows up in your body. If you grind your teeth, brace your muscles, pace the floor, drum your fingers, or tap your feet, you are exhibiting signs of muscular tension.

Sympathetic arousal is a state in which your sympathetic nervous system is keyed up and your body is producing more adrenalin than usual. The sympathetic nervous system controls your heartbeat, breathing, and other automatic activities of your body. When it is aroused, your hands and fingers may feel cold (because adrenalin causes the blood vessels in your fingers to constrict). You also may feel excited or full of anticipation (again due to the increased flow of adrenalin).

These three main types of tension sometimes go together, but not always. Some insomniacs are tense psychologically, though their muscles are relaxed. Others have tense muscles and a calm mind.

Different relaxation techniques may help one form of tension, but not another. If you've tried some kind of relaxation technique and it didn't help, it might be because the type of relaxation you learned did not match the kind of tension you have. Also, relaxation training helps people who are tense—but, paradoxically, causes people who are already relaxed to become frustrated—and makes their sleep worse.

Relaxation techniques can work for relief of both short term and long term insomnia. There was one patient in whom insomnia made a sudden appearance. Cathy O'Hanahan, a 23-year-old mother-to-be, appeared at the clinic in a state of near exhaustion two weeks before her projected time of delivery. She said she hadn't slept for two weeks. She had looked forward to the natural birth of her first baby, but recently her Lamaze teacher had stated that to be ready for natural childbirth, the prospective mothers required plenty of sleep. Immediately, insomnia had struck.

We decided to try relaxation tapes. Mrs. O'Hanahan lay down on the couch, listened to the tape-recorded instructions for the relaxation exercises, and fell asleep before the tape had ended.

She was given a tape to take home and told to do the relaxation exercises whenever she wanted to sleep. Her performance at delivery was no longer threatened, and her insomnia evaporated within two nights.

Elaine Park was an example of how relaxation training can help even a long term sufferer. When she was referred to the sleep disorders center, she had been having trouble getting to sleep at night for two years. Recordings in the sleep lab on three consecutive nights confirmed that she took one and a half to three hours to fall asleep.

According to Mrs. Park, she had been an adequate sleeper until two years earlier, when she had accompanied her husband to a convention in Las Vegas. After an exhausting trip, extended sightseeing, and a night spent gambling, she was unable to fall asleep. She became so worried that something was wrong that she had a week of almost no sleep. The hotel physician prescribed heavy doses of a sedative to restore her for the trip home, and things were better for awhile. But two months later, returning to the United States from a vacation trip in Europe, she again was unable to sleep. She had never heard of jet lag, and her inability to sleep after a high-altitude flight convinced her that something had "snapped" in her nervous system when the airplane was pressurized. Although evaluations at two major medical centers revealed no serious medical problems, she continued to sleep very poorly.

Psychological tests, psychiatric interviews, and 24-hour laboratory observations showed that Mrs. Park was anxious and tense, especially at bedtime. Over a period of two months, she was taught to control her tension through biofeedback and other relaxation techniques. She was told she could take a sleeping pill for one night anytime she experienced more than two nights of insomnia in a row. Gradually, her sleep improved. After nine months, she described only occasional "panic nights," no more than two or three per month, a record with which she was quite satisfied.

These and many other cases show that relaxation techniques at night can help many insomniacs. In fact, they can help *most* insomniacs. The techniques used most often are abdominal breathing, progressive muscle relaxation, meditation, and imaging.

Read through the descriptions that follow and see which one appeals to you. Try it; see how it works. If you don't feel right with it, try another one.

Before You Start

Remember what you learned in the last chapter—*don't try too hard.*
A typical example of trying too hard was an insomniac woman in one
of the center's research projects on biofeedback. She came in for a
series of 15 half-hour sessions and tried to learn relaxation by using
the biofeedback tones. Nothing worked. After 12 sessions, she said "I
can't stand it any longer—I've tried every trick in the book and whatever I try, the tone is high and goes even higher, and the machine
stares in my face and I can't do anything." We asked her to stay
because the project needed 15 sessions, and if she dropped out she
couldn't be used in the study. She agreed to come in for the last three
sessions: "I'll do it, but I'm only going to show up, I'm not going to
try to relax anymore because it's driving me up the wall. I'm just going
to sit there." You can guess the rest of the story. As soon as she was
just sitting there not trying to relax, the tone went down and she
became deeply relaxed.

The idea is not to *try* to relax. You have to let it happen, passively,
especially since you will be using these techniques to help you sleep.
Bedtime is a time to let go.

Relaxation and Stretching Exercises to Do at Night

These soothing exercises take only a few moments, but they can help
melt away both mental stress and muscle tension. First, do them a
few times in the early evening, to get the feel of them, and select those
that really help you relax. Later, you may do them just before you go
to bed or, when you feel particularly tense and find you just cannot
sleep, get out of bed, do them in the dark, and then go back to sleep.
Repeat each exercise several times.

- *The rag-doll dangle.* Stand with your legs apart and bend at the
  waist. Shake your arms and hands loosely. Let your head hang,
  and sway from side to side. Shrug your shoulders. Hang loosely
  for a few moments to relax completely.
- *Head roll.* Drop your chin to your chest. Rotate your head to the
  right and turn your chin to your shoulder. Circle the head back
  and around and over your left shoulder to make a complete
  revolution. Repeat in the opposite direction.

- *Head tilt.* Keep your shoulders down. Tilt the left ear to the left shoulder several times. Tilt the right ear to the right shoulder.
- *Head lift.* Curl your fingers around the sides of your neck, fingers meeting in back. Lift straight upward and forward as though you were trying to lift your head off your shoulders. Turn your head slightly from right to left while you continue lifting.
- *Full body stretch.* Extend your right arm straight up and reach for the ceiling. Reach as high as you can. Pretend you're picking dollar bills off the ceiling. You should feel your entire right side stretch—from the spread-out fingers of your right hand to your right foot. Repeat with your left arm.
- *Torso stretch.* Sit on the edge of the bed with your knees apart, feet on the floor. Hold each end of a hand towel or pillowcase, with your arms stretched out overhead. Holding the towel or pillowcase high, gently stretch out your torso to the left and then to the right.
- *Shoulder stretch.* Still sitting, place your hands on your knees, elbows bent. Press your hands into your knees and lean forward; rotate your shoulders and ribs to the left and then to the right.
- *Do-it-yourself head massage.* Close your eyes and massage your head and neck in firm, small circles. With your head and neck limp, massage the skull, then massage down along the neck vertebrae to the shoulder. (If you have a partner, you can go limp and let him or her give you a full head and body massage.)
- *Back stretch.* Lie flat on your back in bed. Push your spine into the bed, flattening your back and pulling in your abdomen. Release, go limp in all muscles, and breathe deeply. Repeat several times. Remain limp and breathe deeply.

Mind Games to Use When You Go to Bed

These are techniques to use at bedtime, especially if you are overly alert and tense. They should help you drift off to sleep.

- *Be a sponge.* Lie on your back, completely relaxed, and imagine you are a sponge, arms limp and away from the body, shoulders relaxed, legs apart and loose. Press your neck and back into the bed. Close your eyes, and breathe deeply through your nose. Let each part of your body relax, while thinking of your body as a sponge, limp, soaking up peace and tranquility from the universe around you.

- *The sighing breath.* Inhale deeply through the nostrils, then with lips puckered (as if cooling soup), exhale very slowly through the mouth for as long as you can. Concentrate on the long, sighing sound and feel the tension dissolve.
- *Counting.* Close your eyes and let your body go limp. Let yourself sink deep into comfort. Count slowly from one hundred down to zero, visualizing the numbers being written very slowly and carefully and beautifully. See them in downward progression, as if each successive number were standing one step lower on a staircase. Feel the relaxation spread through every muscle and nerve of your body as you see the numbers. Or you can pretend that you are slowly and carefully drawing each number on a huge blackboard or across a giant sky, drawing each number as large as possible. Continue until sleep takes over.
- *Creating pictures.* Think of a pleasant and restful scene. You can picture a simple object—study every line of it, appreciating its graceful curves, texture, and feel. Or picture one color in a variety of patterns and hues, continually blending and changing. Or picture an entire scene with a quiet mood: a silent, white snow scene with soft snowflakes falling slowly or a pastoral painting of greens and blues, with cows and horses contentedly grazing along a meadow. Or imagine that you're lying on the beach in the warm sun. Try to actually experience the scene, not just watch it. Feel the sun on your back, your toes squishing in the sand, the breeze blowing on your skin. Perhaps you can hear a bird in the background, smell the clear air, or smell the moss in the nearby woods. On the other hand, if the details distract you, don't worry about them. Just experience lying in the sun being warm.

Many people like to imagine themselves floating. Envision yourself floating on a cloud, or on an air mattress floating on a warm, gentle sea, with the water surrounding you and supporting you.

One of the best ways to relax is to think of downward movement. Picture yourself floating down like a leaf, or imagine going down a staircase or riding down an escalator. The lower you go, the deeper you go into relaxation and sleep.

Abdominal Breathing

One of the easiest relaxation exercises to start with—and one that works with many kinds of tension—is the simple technique of abdominal breathing. But don't start doing it at bedtime until you really know how to do it. Start by practicing it in the daytime or early in the evening. Only after you are skilled can you use it to make you sleepy in bed.

At first glance, the technique seems so simple that you might think you need no practice at all. You want the technique to become almost automatic, however, so that when you go to sleep, you don't have to control it but can just drift off to sleep; so practice for at least two weeks, every day for 20 minutes.

You will know you are getting good at abdominal breathing when you become so relaxed doing it that you almost (or even do) fall asleep. Or you can tell you're getting good if you get feelings of heaviness, lightness, or warmth; a feeling of floating or of butterflies in the stomach; or some other strange sensation. Surprisingly, many insomniacs initially experience these feelings as unpleasant, but as you learn to recognize them for the signs of good relaxation, they will become pleasant. Once those sensations come, and when the relaxation is almost automatic, you can use abdominal breathing when you want to go to sleep at bedtime or in the middle of the night.

However, you should use abdominal breathing only once during the night. If you are having a poor night because you drank too much coffee or because a cold is coming on, for example, and you keep trying to use abdominal breathing and it doesn't get you to sleep, the technique gets associated with frustration and failure. What you need to do is use the technique once for a half hour or so. If it doesn't work, don't keep using it that same night.

Here's how to do abdominal breathing: Lie down and notice your breathing—the rhythm and the depth. Don't try to change it, just breathe normally. After you have observed the rhythm, then start to breathe more with your abdomen and less with your chest. (Put one hand on your abdomen and the other on your chest to feel that the abdomen goes up and down, but the chest doesn't.) Don't breathe deeper, or slower, or faster; just keep the same rhythm, but breathe with your abdomen. It may feel funny at first, because you've been told all your life not to stick your stomach out—and here you are trying to make your stomach go up and down. If it doesn't come easily, it may help to put your hands behind your head—this helps to stop your chest breathing. (If your chest moves a little bit, it's okay.) Or you can put a book or even a heavier weight on your stomach and make it go up and down. You can breathe through your mouth or nose, whichever is comfortable. If you are uncomfortable, you probably are breathing too slowly and your body isn't getting enough oxygen. If you are getting a little dizzy, you are breathing too fast, getting too much oxygen.

When you are comfortable with this much, the next step is to change the breathing just a little bit more. After each outbreath, stop for a half a second or so and think about the breath you just took. Was it smooth? Was it comfortable? Appreciate each breath for itself.

In . . . out, pause; in . . . out, pause.

Some people need to practice for ten minutes and they have it, and others need to practice for a month before it feels comfortable.

Once the abdominal breathing and the pause feel comfortable, go to the next step: As you breathe, feel the air on your upper lip or inside your nose—anywhere you can feel the air come in and out. Some people feel the movement of the air, others feel the spot get warmer with exhalation and cooler with inhalation. Search for the place where you feel the breathing best. When you have found it, concentrate on that spot. Concentrate totally. Feel the fresh air come in and the old air go out. From now on when you do abdominal breathing, after you have your breathing organized, focus on that spot and feel the air going in and out. Once you get the feel of doing all this, it will let you really relax.

Sometimes a thought will intrude as you focus on your breathing. If you find your mind wandering, don't simply push the thought away, because it will come back. Instead, take the thought and imagine writing it on a piece of paper. Then imagine having a balloon; roll up the paper with the thought on it, tie it to the string of the balloon, and let the balloon go. Don't get angry when a thought comes, simply accept that you are thinking about a phone call, a yellow elephant, or whatever; write it down on a piece of paper; roll it up; tie it to the balloon; and let it go. Then see the thought with the balloon drift up into the sky. When it is high enough, return your attention to your breathing and continue to concentrate on the air coming in and going out.

Sometimes your mind is so abuzz with thoughts that you can't make the balloons fast enough and there just is no way to concentrate on the breathing spot. That may be the time for you simply to stop practicing for that session and go take care of one of the things you are thinking of, or do something else.

Some people say that if the mind is too full, it helps to find a two syllable word to focus on. (But don't use the word "relax." For some reason, it makes many people tense. "Relax" is not a relaxing word.) Find your own special word, like "deep-down" "serene," "heavy," "tranquil," or "floating." Use one syllable when you breathe in, one syllable when you breathe out. Or you can use two words, like "calm, warm"—or "cool, warm" if you want to tie it in with the temperature in your nose. Say these words to yourself with each breath for awhile, until your mind calms down.

In India, they practice abdominal breathing for months, so if it doesn't work right away, don't give up. You couldn't ride a bicycle in the first two minutes, either. You have to practice each day, probably for a few weeks.

Advanced Relaxation Techniques

For these techniques, you probably will need the help of a professional, since very few people can learn them well enough to be effective without some instruction.

Biofeedback

With biofeedback, you can learn to control some of your body's activities by monitoring body function on a machine that uses meters, sounds, or lights to tell you the moment-by-moment physiological state of muscle tension, skin temperature, heart rate, blood pressure, or other things. You observe the natural changes that occur, then you learn which mental states go with these changes. Soon, you usually are able to influence functions that you previously did not have any control over, and you can make yourself relax or tense at will, without the machine. This technique is especially good for muscle tension and sympathetic arousal.

Biofeedback is like a mirror that shows you what one of your body functions does so that you can learn how to influence it. For example, if somebody offered you $10,000 to wiggle your ears right now, you probably couldn't do it. The proper muscles and nerves are there, but you don't know how to give them the signal to work. If you wanted that $10,000 badly enough, you might stand in front of a mirror and try all kinds of contortions to make your ears wiggle. Probably, at first, none of them would work—then suddenly, your ears would move just a little. Not really knowing how you did it, you'd try it again and again. Finally, after a few days in front of the mirror, you'd learn how to do it.

In the same way, biofeedback can be like a mirror. It can measure, say, the muscle tension in your forehead (or other places) and tell you when your muscles are tense or relaxed. Usually, the machine uses a tone that goes up and down to give you this information. When the tone goes up, you know that you are getting more tense. When the tone goes down, you know that your muscles are relaxing. By self-exploration, you find out what makes tension go up and down and learn how to be more relaxed.

Biofeedback also can work by measuring other body variables, such as finger temperature. However, it is harder to learn to warm your fingers than to relax your muscles, because your finger does not warm up until you've been relaxed for a minute or more, whereas muscle tension registers on the machine immediately.

When you are relaxed, your hand and finger temperature is usually in the 90s. If the temperature is in the 70s (and you do not suffer from poor circulation), you may have sympathetic-arousal tension and would probably benefit from doing temperature biofeedback, either on your own or with a biofeedback therapist.

You can do an at-home version of temperature biofeedback if you want to try it. Take a room thermometer, tape it to your finger, and measure the temperature. Then do one of the relaxation techniques, such as abdominal breathing, for about five minutes. Look at the thermometer again and see if the temperature has risen a little. If it has, whatever you did was relaxing. Do more of it. If it hasn't risen in about five minutes, whatever you did didn't help you relax. So try something else.

Sometimes, tension is caused by the *content* of what you're thinking about—the beach versus the office. Sometimes, it's more *how* you think: You can think about something in a relaxed way or you can think about it with your mind and body tensed.

You may have to discover a new state of mind. Some people don't really know what "relaxation" is. What they think of as relaxing is more like anxiously waiting for a taxi to come. If you are one of these people, you may have to experience and recognize an entirely new state. Biofeedback can help you do this.

· · · ● ● · · ·

At Dartmouth Medical School, I did a biofeedback study on 45 insomniacs. They kept Sleep Logs at home and spent three nights in the laboratory before biofeedback, after several weeks of biofeedback, and nine months later. The study showed that relaxation through biofeedback clearly helped tense and anxious insomniacs, but did not help people who were already muscularly relaxed but still could not sleep.

Then I did another biofeedback study on 16 very serious insomniacs—people whose insomnia had been relentless for at least two years and who showed insomnia on home Sleep Logs for at least 8 out of 14 nights. Patients were again evaluated for 3 nights in the Dartmouth Sleep Disorders Center, by a battery of psychological questionnaires and by interview, then received biofeedback training at our lab and at the laboratory of Dr. Ernest Hartmann in Boston.

Both studies showed that biofeedback can have a long-lasting effect on insomnia. Sleep improved after the biofeedback and was still improved at follow-up nine months later. This finding is heartening, because in many other conditions, biofeedback training seems to have only a temporary effect. However, remember that muscle-tension biofeedback works only in insomniacs whose muscles are tense when they're trying to sleep.

· · ● ● ● · ·

Sometimes, relaxation training with biofeedback can be helpful even in crisis situations. Mrs. Belle Wells went through a very difficult divorce at about the same time that one of her three children developed leukemia and died. Then, a month later, her only sister was killed in a car accident. In addition, finances forced her to remain at home to take care of her other two small children. She was under extreme stress and, not surprisingly, suffered from severe insomnia. It took her about two hours to fall asleep each night, and she also suffered from many long awakenings throughout the night. Lab examination showed that Mrs. Wells' forehead muscle tension was extremely high, during both wakefulness and sleep, and she was nervous and agitated.

She was enrolled in a course of biofeedback training and was taught how to relax her forehead before bedtime. She also used the technique during the day. When she found herself racing about and losing control, she stopped for a few seconds of relaxation and then got on with her work. She gradually started to master her situation, and follow-up records in the sleep lab nine months later showed almost totally normal sleep.

Meditation

Meditation produces a state of passive concentration, sometimes called an *alpha state* because the brain puts out alpha waves, as it does in the last moments before falling asleep. This quiet state of inner reflection is beneficial for people who are psychologically tense or have sympathetic arousal. Meditation helps to decrease the activity of the sympathetic nervous system and thus helps to reduce tension and anxiety, slow respiration and heart rate, and lower blood pressure. If you ever were completely relaxed and centered within yourself, you probably experienced something like meditation.

There are many ways to meditate. Some, such as Transcendental Meditation (TM), involve concentrating on a *mantra* (a word or phrase). Other methods include concentrating on your breathing, as in yoga or Zen meditation, or focusing your gaze on a lighted candle, a leaf, or still water. Each technique is designed to produce a sense of calmness and inner harmony that wipes away tension.

You need to learn meditation from a trainer or guide. To find out about classes in your area, check the yellow pages under "Meditation," check for classes at universities or local YMCAs, or ask a minister, priest, or rabbi.

Autogenic Training

Autogenic training is a procedure that involves repeating the same phrases over and over, while concentrating on feelings of heaviness and warmth. Through suggestion, the "heavy" muscles relax, and the "warm" flesh receives better circulation.

You start by thinking the phrase, "My right arm is heavy," repeating it several times. Then you go to other areas of your body. Later, you continue with "My arms are warm," "My legs are warm," "My entire body is warm."

In a 1968 experiment, Dr. Michael Kahn, then at Yale, Bruce Baker at Harvard, and Jay Weiss at Rockefeller University taught 16 insomniac college students to use autogenic training. At the end of the experiment, the students had cut their average time needed to fall asleep from 52 to 22 minutes. These results were matched in 1974 by Dr. Richard Bootzin at Northwestern University in Chicago, who found that a month's daily practice of either progressive relaxation or autogenic training produced 50 percent improvement in falling asleep.

Autogenic training is not a method that can be learned in a few minutes. It should be learned from a competent teacher over several weeks or months to gain maximum effect.

Progressive Relaxation

When a muscle has been tense for a few seconds, its natural tendency is to relax. Progressive relaxation (PR) uses this fact. You tense different muscle groups in the body and then let them go, to experience how a relaxed muscle feels. Later, you should be able to reestablish that feeling of relaxation without having to tense your muscles first.

You can test whether PR might be useful to you. Sit down in a comfortable chair or lie on your bed. Take a few comfortable breaths. Now focus your attention on your right hand. Make a fist with that hand, and tighten it as hard as you can. White knuckles! Tense, tense! Keep it tense for about five or six seconds. Then let go, open the fist, and let the muscles do what they want. Observe how your hand feels. Whatever the muscles in your hand do now, let them do more of it. Observe the hand for about 20 or 30 seconds. Then repeat the exercise. Make a tight fist again. Tense! White knuckles! After about six seconds or so, let go. Observe your hand again as it relaxes. Let it do more of whatever it is doing right now. Then compare your right hand, which is now deeply relaxed, with your left hand, which is in its normal state. Do you perceive any difference? That is the difference between your usual state and a deeply relaxed state.

If you felt a marked difference between the two hands when you relaxed the second time, you are a good candidate for progressive relaxation training. Basically, you will learn to work the various muscle groups in your body, tensing and relaxing each of them twice and observing them as they relax. You might try this on your own. After the right hand, you would tense the right arm, then the left hand and the left arm. Then you go to your face, tensing the muscles in your forehead and around your eyes, then the cheeks, lips, the muscles in your neck, the shoulders, the abdominal muscles, the buttocks, thighs, the calves, and the feet. (For the feet, pull your toes up and spread them out, because pulling them down and tensing them can lead to cramps.)

Don't rush. Take your time. Tense the muscle for several seconds and observe each relaxation for 20 to 30 seconds.

If any of the tensing gives you pain or cramps, do the exercise once more, but with less intensity. The important thing is that you notice the feeling that gets into each muscle group once you let it relax.

Do progressive relaxation for the first week or two in the late afternoon or early evening, not at the time when you want to go to sleep. Be prepared to experience some of the same unusual feelings that you might feel with abdominal breathing: heaviness, lightness, warmth, feelings of floating, butterflies in the stomach. Also, when one is deeply relaxed, sometimes the body twitches. Let the twitches happen. Sometimes, all kinds of emotions may flood through your mind. Tears may come to your eyes, or you might feel very excited, or just heavy and leaden. Let these feelings wash over you without letting them frighten you away from relaxation. Usually, as you continue to relax, they will disappear. If not, it might be time to talk to a professional about them, because they might be important indicators of why it's so difficult for you to relax.

When you are really good at this technique, eliminate the tensing phase. Simply make mental contact with each muscle group and let the muscles experience the same degree of relaxation that comes over them naturally after tensing. This is how to use the technique most effectively as a sleep inducer.

Neurolinguistic Programming

Neurolinguistic Programming (NLP) is a relatively new technique that hasn't been clinically tested yet by the sleep profession. It is a sort of mirror image of body language: By putting your body into the sensations, feelings and positions of a past successful experience, you program your brain to be able to repeat that experience. It sounds complicated, but once instructed in it, many people find it quite a powerful and effective tool.

It would work like this for helping you fall asleep better: When you get into bed, think about a time when you fell asleep very easily. Remember a specific time and go back and experience it in your imagination. Do you see a picture? What position were you in? Did you hear anything? Were you thinking anything in particular? What was it that caused you to be comfortable and sleepy? Did you have a certain feeling or emotion? Once you reexperience what made you sleep well before, you can use these same words, positions, pictures, or feelings now to help put you into a sleepy state.

Choosing a Technique

We have guided you through a number of relaxation techniques. There are many others. Some people relax deeply when they are in deep prayer. Others learn self-hypnosis or get into a relaxed state through Hatha yoga.

We do not expect you to become proficient in all methods of relaxation. But if tension is a problem at bedtime, we do recommend that you choose one of the methods we have described, or some other method you know about, and then practice it. It is important that whatever method you use, you learn it thoroughly. You want the method to be automatic and natural, so that—without using any energy to direct it—you can just let it happen.

···· 8 ····

Learn to Manage Your Stress All Day

John Remington was a social worker with a private welfare agency in one of our large inner cities. He enjoyed his job, and there was much to do. Clients needed help finding their way around the system and advice on how to apply for jobs, food stamps, or welfare. Others simply needed to talk—to get a pat on the back, encouragement to carry on, help to work out a marital conflict. There was a need to organize teenagers and get them off the street. People with legal problems needed help. There was much adversity—from landlords who did not want their renters to file petitions with the city, from politicians who wanted everything swept under the rug, from drug dealers who felt John could be a threat.

John was married and had two preschool children. His family, too, needed attention and nurturance. He did not make as much money as he would had he worked in a government job, so he tried to compensate by doing much of the remodeling work around his home himself. Every time he spent an evening at home, he knew that some of his clients at work would be disappointed. So he tried to stretch himself, hurrying home for dinner and two hours with his family, then running back for another three hours at his job. He became irritable and moody and started to sleep very poorly.

John's case is typical of many insomniacs. As we said in Chapter 2, about half of all cases of insomnia are related to psychological problems—anxiety, depression, tension—that often are brought on by a bad marriage, loneliness, an overly demanding job, or other emotionally related conditions. On top of that are the stresses of society.

Our cities are crowded; the traffic is terrible; crime is rampant; drug use surrounds us; and we read daily of corruption, war, and a world that is rapidly being destroyed by overpopulation and pollution.

You go all day, busy, your problems seething inside you—then night comes and all those things run through your mind over and over. You try to relax when you go to bed, but you can't; your brain is still in turmoil, working. A troubled mind almost always means troubled sleep or no sleep at all.

When you are confronted with stress, your adrenalin goes up, your heart beats faster, your blood pressure rises, and your muscles tense. These body changes are good for an emergency reaction—such as fighting a saber-toothed tiger or running from a brushfire—but most of our stresses are slow burning, lasting for months or years: how to get along with your spouse or teenage kid or boss. You cannot deal with these stresses using an emergency reaction designed to last ten minutes, but your body still reacts as if you could. The system designed for the short fight-flight reaction breaks down. People often develop headaches, ulcers, or sexual problems—but most often, they develop insomnia.

Sometimes, the connection between stress and insomnia is obvious. Insomnia comes after you have had an argument with someone you love, your boss has criticized you for something that wasn't your fault, or you have been trying to make a deadline that you know is impossible. Or you may have "Christmas Eve insomnia" on exciting occasions. Remember how you lay awake as a child on Christmas Eve? As adults, we may be just as excited the night before starting a job, making a big presentation, or leaving for a vacation.

Also, events in the evening can carry over into sleep. Laboratory studies show that when people watch horror films or other emotionally disturbing films before bedtime, they frequently carry the disturbing events into their sleep and dreams.

At other times, the stress connection is subtle. A *long term* problem may be causing tension and insomnia, wearing away at you without your realizing it, eroding your self-esteem and building your anger, tension, or frustration.

Many patients honestly don't feel that they have a stress-connected problem. Others repress it: "I don't have a mental problem. I just can't sleep." And they simply take more sleeping pills instead of dealing with the mental pain caused by the tension and stress. Or they overeat, drink, or smoke to relieve the anxiety—all of which can add to the insomnia.

Even if people realize that stress is involved, they may not know how to delve into the problem and deal with it. Consciously or unconsciously, they avoid their problem instead of finding what is stressing them and working out ways to deal with it. Sometimes you can change what is stressing you, and sometimes you can't. But even just knowing that tension could be the cause of your insomnia can help.

Research shows that it often is not the big problems—such as divorce or the death of a close friend—that drag us down, but the small, irritating, daily hassles. And often, it isn't the stressful situation itself that causes the problem, but our attitude toward the situation and our reaction to it. We don't have to meet minor happenings as though they were major crises, but we often do.

You can sometimes reduce stress by changing how you look at things. A burned dinner, spilled milk, a flat tire, a bill unpaid, a job lost, a child crying—all are potentially stressful situations. How much they affect you depends on how you react to them. Dr. Albert Ellis, founder of the Institute for Rational Emotive Therapy in New York, claims that "awfulizing"—reacting to everything as if it were the worst catastrophe—is at the root of many psychological problems.

Often, we are more in control of our destinies than we give ourselves credit for. We can make other choices: We can choose to drive to work by a slower but less congested route. We can choose not to go to a party where we are sure we won't like the people. We can choose to pack a bag lunch and sit in the park instead of gulping a hot dog or burger on the run. We can choose to drop annoying, nonproductive activities, and we can even choose not to associate with a negative person in our lives who may be dragging us down.

Check Yourself for Hidden Tension

Could you be tenser than you think you are? Most of us are unaware that stress and tension are getting to us, and it's important to have a way to check ourselves throughout the day.

Check yourself right now and again during the day whenever you think of it—especially when you are anxious, are working hard at a problem, or find that you are tight and hurrying for no good reason.

Here are the tension clues to look for:

- Tight neck or jaw muscles
- Tight shoulders or back
- Jutted-out chin
- Gritting or grinding of teeth
- Tight, strained voice
- Hunched shoulders
- Tightly curled toes or fingers, drumming with your fingers
- Foot tapping, legs constantly in motion
- Rigid spine
- Tight forehead muscles, sometimes with a headache
- Sweating hands, feet, or armpits
- Irritability, overreacting to small things
- Frowning
- High pulse rate, heart pounding rapidly
- Brusque, jerky movements with muscles tight or braced
- Irregular, shallow breathing or sighing respiration
- Feeling of suffocation
- Nervous stomach, cramping, or nausea
- Urinating frequently
- Smoking intensely
- Fluttering eyes or eyestrain

When you feel any of these signs coming on, take several deep breaths, try to smile, not just with your lips but also with your eyes, and let your muscles relax. You don't *have* to grip the phone grimly when you talk, pound your feet when you walk, or rush headlong, harried and hurried, through the housework. Slow your voice, slow your walk, relax the fingers holding a pencil or telephone, and ease your mind and body into a relaxed approach to whatever you are doing.

Even when there is no way to eliminate stress from a job or social situation, you can learn to stop in the middle of a crisis and mentally check for tight muscles and tension. The very act of checking often helps you relax. And try to smile with your eyes even in the middle of a crisis. It is surprising how you can smile with your mouth and still be tense, but when you try smiling with your eyes, tension melts.

It is not always easy to remember to check. A good way to get into the habit is to buy self-adhesive red dots and glue them to some places where you look occasionally, such as the top drawer of your

desk, the refrigerator, or the dashboard of your car. Everytime you
see a red dot, stop and check for the signs of tension. Ask yourself,
"Am I in control?" Move whatever muscles are tight, take two comfortable breaths, smile to yourself, and go on.

You can develop your own ways to help ease tension. President
Kennedy used to lean back on the wall, close his eyes, and relax
completely whenever free moments came, even the few minutes in
an elevator. Dr. Paul Dudley White rode his bike and walked. One
famous network science editor hums before going on the air. A surgeon
friend sings to relax himself before he operates.

Take Control

One of the most important recent insights in psychology is that it isn't
the stress of hard work that gets us into trouble, it's being in a situation
over which we have no control. It's the frustration, anxiety, and tension
of being unable to do something about a situation that needs changing.

People who can't sleep most often are those who have family or
job problems that they feel they have no control over. But there often
is a way to fix such problems, if we only give ourselves time to reason
and think about them logically. Here's how.

Worry Time

If you're the kind of insomniac who lies in bed with thoughts buzzing
through your head, and you can't stop them, or you find yourself
worrying about finances or your job or feel that you are losing control,
Worry Time might be the solution for you.

Here's how Worry Time works: Sometime during the evening,
long before you go to bed, schedule a half hour to do the work of
worry so you don't have to do it in bed. To do your worrying, go into
a quiet room and tell your family not to bother you, not even for
telephone calls. Take 30 or 40 blank 3- by 5-inch file cards and a
pencil with you. Just sit and relax. Pretty soon, if you're a worrier or
concerned about losing control, worries will start buzzing around. As
they come, write each one down on one of the cards. They don't have
to be important worries; they can be dumb worries or little worries.
No matter, whatever bothersome thought comes into your head, it
gets a separate card. You'll find that this helps immediately, because

anything written down doesn't buzz in your head so much. Sit there and do that for perhaps 15 or 20 minutes—until you can't come up with any more worries.

Sometime, you may just sit there and the worries don't come. For half an hour, there is no worry buzzing around in your mind. That's okay—you've simply used this time to relax. So don't sit there and worry that you might not have any worries!

The second step is to make categories of the worries. This establishes some order into the chaos and starts putting the worries under your control.

You might have one batch of worries about your finances, another batch about your relationships, and another about how you aren't any good—whatever. But don't make too many categories; usually, from three to seven is about right. If you have a category for each worry, then you haven't done anything.

Some people classify their worries by content, others by how important the worry is—there are little worries, big worries, stupid worries, etc. It doesn't matter how you classify them, as long as the categories suit your situation.

Once you have them in groups, think about each group carefully and see what you can do with the worries in that group. At the bottom of each card, write down what seems to be the best solution. For example, if a worry is that tomorrow you have too much to do, that card should contain a possible outline of your schedule for the next day. If a worry is that you are going to forget important telephone calls tomorrow, write down all the calls that you have to make and use that card for your calls tomorrow morning. If a worry is that you have only $200 left in the bank and you have $800 worth of bills to pay, decide right then which bills to pay and which bills not to pay, who you have to call to explain, perhaps to make partial payment, and just how you're going to manage the problem.

The trick is that the solution has to be written down, not just kept in your head. If it is written down, it helps you let the worry go. It is a written contract with yourself to carry out the solutions. The next day, you do the things on your cards.

Of course, there are some worries that you have absolutely no control over. You simply can't do anything about them. In that case, write down, "I will not deal with this worry today" or "This worry is out of my control" or "I will deal with that in three weeks when so-and-so comes to town." Sometimes, there may be a person who is causing you distress, but your conclusion is that you cannot change that person's personality. You might think of what you could say to them the next time you see them, or you could write down, "I have done everything I can; the ball is in the other person's court, and now I have to wait until it comes back."

The goal is to face each worry squarely and decide what or whether you are going to do something about it—so that, at the end of your session, you have each worry processed in some way. Put the cards away to look at in the morning. You have done your work of worrying. And if worries now come to you in the middle of the night, you can say, "I dealt with that last night, the solution is settled. Go away."

Sometimes, though rarely, there will be worries that don't come during Worry Time, but come later on. It's not a bad idea to have a card near your bed—then you can put that worry onto its card to be dealt with the next evening. Sometimes, a solution doesn't work and a worry comes back night after night. In that case, perhaps your solution wasn't right. Think it through again, or perhaps see a counselor.

The main idea is to have your worries thought about before you go to bed and when you are still thinking clearly—so you don't make mountains out of molehills in the middle of the night when the stupidest little worries can drive you crazy. Now you can say, "It's okay, not to worry, I know what to do." Worrying about problems in the middle of the night not only can enlarge the problem, but you can't do anything about it then. There are a lot of worries that you can't deal with at three o'clock in the morning that *can* be dealt with at eight in the evening. For example, if your worry is that you forgot your mother's birthday, you can call. If your worry is that "I'm not getting along with my son too well," if he is still up doing his homework, maybe you can go in and talk to him.

Schedule a Worry Time every night or every other night for a week, maybe two. If it helps, continue doing it. If it doesn't work, give it up. Some people choose not to do Worry Time regularly, but only when their problems become hectic and bothersome.

A variation on Worry Time that works well is called The Worst Possible Scenario. When you get to the analysis of the cards and the various alternatives, ask yourself, "What is the worst thing that can happen?" Then ask yourself whether you could stand it. No matter how serious the situation, you can use this technique to put things in perspective: "If I stand up for this principle at my job, what is the worst thing that could happen? Probably, that my boss would fire me." Can you handle that, and is the principle worth that consequence? If it is, then go for it. If you would not be able to handle it or it isn't worth getting fired, make a different decision. In either case, you no longer have to worry about it.

It usually turns out that the worries are not really that bad once you face them. What you are worrying about may not even happen— but if they do, you are ready.

Reducing Tension and Coping with Stress

Anytime things get too bad to handle, think about the fact that you don't need to have a frenzied, tense, anxious reaction to life. You can learn to respond differently. Read through the following suggestions and mark those that might apply to you. Go through the list again and put another mark next to the ones you would like to do something about. Then choose the *one thing* most applicable to you that you would like to work on right away. (You can always go back and work on the others later.)

- Think about what you really want from life. List some specific goals for the next few months and for longer into the future. Try to devote as much time as possible to these goals and to major problems, rather than to trivia.
- Organize your day for the things you really want or need to do, so that you are not always in a frenzy, struggling against time. Keep lists for shopping and for things you want to do. Carry a notebook for jotting down notes as you think of things. In the evening, look at your lists and engagement calendar and plan your coming day.
- Use small bits of time. Watch only the television programs that are really important to you. Use an hour in the evening for a family hobby or to get a small job done. Carry a book to read, letters to write, or other small projects with you, so that you can take advantage of any waiting or commuting time.
- Get help for the less important jobs you can afford to delegate. Learn how to say no to things you don't really want or need to do. Eliminate unnecessary tasks. Simplify.

- Learn to concentrate on a task when you do it. Don't let your mind wander to other problems while you're taking care of the current one. Create an environment that promotes peace. Try to eliminate distracting noises and conflicting activities, so that you can concentrate on what you are doing.
- Try to calm your sense of urgency. You don't have to rush through each day as if you're running a race. Take a deep breath, hum a tune, and walk a little slower.
- When something worries you, talk it out. Don't bottle it up. Talk to your family or a friend. If that isn't enough, consider professional help.
- Allow time for self-contemplation and thinking. Many people find that exploring their religion more deeply or reading the great philosophers gives them a sense of purpose and peace that helps put oil on the waters of stressful situations.
- Try to find work you really like. Remember, it isn't the stress of work that wears us out, but the stress of frustration and failure. Working long hours or doing hard physical labor rarely leads to dangerous tension. But there *is* a relationship between anxiety and lack of job satisfaction. If you are tense because you feel inadequate at your job, take some courses or read books to improve your skills. Two big causes of stress on the job are not knowing what is expected and not having adequate facts or tools. Perhaps you could solve such problems through a friendly discussion with your boss.
- How much energy are you putting into being scared? Into being angry? Try cooperation instead of competition and anger. You don't always have to edge out the other person on the highway or win an argument. Learn to recognize and stop destructive, angry feelings.
- Do something physical. If you feel pent-up anger or frustration, cool off by jogging, doing heavy gardening, or working out. Take a walk, hit a golf or tennis ball, go to a dance, or go for a swim. Exercise reduces tension.
- Escape for a while. Go to a movie, visit a friend, or play a game with your child. Then come back and deal with your difficulty. (But don't keep escaping; learn to deal with problems as promptly as you can.)

- When you relax, really relax. Some people watch TV or lie on a beach and still are tense. Put your problem out of your mind and lose yourself to relaxing.
- Enjoy your family. Whether it's with your parents, your spouse, or your children, you can gain understanding and support as well as enjoyment.
- If boredom or loneliness is your problem, build some variety and laughter into your life. Arrange time for play and time for intimacy. Bring positive energies into your life; filter out negative energies. Join some new groups, volunteer to help solve a problem in your area. Learn to laugh—go to a funny movie, watch some funny television shows, read a funny book, try to make some new friends who are positive and have a sense of humor.

You Are Allowed to Be Imperfect

Give the best of your efforts and ability, but don't feel guilty if you can't achieve the impossible. Learn to be a perfectionist on the important things, not on low-priority items.

The drive for perfection has been called "role-model stress" by one researcher. In women, it may arise from trying to do it all—be a perfect mother and wife and have a successful career and a full social life. In men, it may arise from the feeling that one must never admit grief, failure, defeat, frustration, or that things are going badly.

Our fantasies and dreams don't always turn out in real life. We all have problems, and it's through these problems that we are challenged to grow. You're going to make mistakes and have failures—it happens to even the most successful people.

You Are Not Stuck

When you are in a frenzy, you need to stop and reassess, to sit down alone and contemplate your own personal issues. Decide what is not going right, and make some guesses as to how it could be fixed. Most people simply assume that they are stuck and have no way out. That's seldom true. Read through our ideas or come up with some of your own. Select some rational alternatives and try one. If the outcome is not what you expect, it's probably not irreversible. You can always go back to your former way of doing things if the new way is not working—or try another idea.

You also can withdraw from your world for a mental break once or twice a day. If at all possible, put your feet up, close your eyes, breathe slowly and deeply, and relax your muscles. Take a three-minute vacation to Tahiti by imagining yourself lying on a beach in the sun, or use some of the relaxation techniques we described in Chapter 7. A relaxation break is a three-minute vacation you can take every day of the year.

If you have tried all these things and nothing seems to work, if you feel that tension and stress are your major problems and you just can't seem to solve them, it may be time to get some professional help to get you started on the right road. Check with your doctor, a psychologist, a psychiatrist, a local clinic, a university, or even the telephone book for instruction in biofeedback, time management, and other techniques for reducing stress that you think are appropriate for you. Some companies now offer stress-reduction workshops for their employees.

Even though it often is difficult to make changes in lifestyle, the effort is worth it. Exchanging stress and tension for a sense of control can lift a heavy weight from your shoulders and give you a feeling of security and tranquility. The more you can master your life during the day, the more likely it is that your night time sleep will become sound and satisfying again.

··· 9 ···

Make Your Diet Work For Your Sleep

American Indians used nutmeg oil to encourage sleep. A traditional German formula is ground anise and honey in warm milk, or valerian or chamomile tea. Swiss villagers grow melissa (lemon balm) in their gardens; in England, cowslips are brewed into a bedtime tea. Your grandmother might have recommended a glass of warm milk.

There is solid research evidence that your sleep may be affected by what you eat. Dr. Nathaniel Kleitman, the University of Chicago sleep pioneer, compared the effects on sleep of a variety of bedtime snacks. He and his colleagues found that a glass of milk, Ovaltine (made from milk and cereal), or Horlicks (a Scotch malt drink) before retiring did help people to sleep. In 1969, Dr. J. W. Fara and his colleagues found that cats sleep better when they have milk or fat in their stomachs. In 1975, Dr. F. Phillips and his coworkers at St. George's Hospital in London found that differences in the amount of carbohydrate and fat in the diet had an effect on the relative proportions of delta (deep) sleep and REM (dreaming) sleep. Dr. Harris Lieberman, of the Massachusetts Institute of Technology, showed that subjects had slower reaction times and were sleepier after a high-starch lunch than after a high-protein lunch.

In this chapter, we will discuss the latest nutritional advice for insomniacs. Approach this advice in the same way as you do other parts of this program: Be your own sleep therapist. Change your diet and see what happens to your sleep. Allow at least a week for results, since your body needs time to make adjustments.

Your General Diet

No matter what other factors are involved, you'll sleep better if you're healthy. One of the keys to being healthy is your general diet. The guidelines to good eating are simple if you remember a few key points.

(These guidelines, by the way, follow the findings and advice of the American Heart Association, the recent Surgeon General's and Department of Agriculture's recommendations on diet, and the recommendations of the American Cancer Society, as well as our own clinical findings—so if you follow this advice, your diet also should help protect you against heart disease, high blood pressure, diabetes, cancer, obesity and other problems.

Diet *can* make a difference for the person with insomnia. People on diets without proper nutrients have been found to suffer from insomnia as well as from fatigue, irritability, tension, depression, and other problems. There can be physical as well as psychological problems when your diet contains inadequate amounts of vitamins, minerals, and other nutrients.

Make your food count. If you're going to take in calories, try to take in nutrients, too.

Rule 1. Eat lots of salads and fresh vegetables.

Whenever possible, avoid prepackaged, precooked, and chemical-filled foods, such as TV dinners. Develop a taste for fresh, unprocessed foods as they come from the earth—from "A" for asparagus to "Z" for zucchini.

To get the most nutritional benefit, buy vegetables fresh, store them for as short a time as possible, and don't overcook them. Steamed vegetables, still a little firm and crunchy, have more vitamins than overcooked, soggy ones. Eating leftover vegetables in a salad is better than reheating them a second or third time.

Rule 2. Eat lots of whole grains and fiber foods.

Instead of eating sugared cereal, pie, cake, and white bread, get complex carbohydrates from potatoes, fruits, salads, vegetables, whole-grain breads, and unsweetened cereals. This is likely to reduce your risk of heart disease, diabetes, and even certain types of cancers such as cancer of the colon. It also is likely to lower cholesterol and triglyceride levels, reduce high blood pressure, and improve digestion. And the many B vitamins in whole grains are good for calming irritability and tension, which often cause insomnia.

Rule 3. Eat a variety of foods.

The body needs more than 50 nutrients for optimal health. No single food contains all the essential nutrients, so it is important to eat a *variety* of foods. In addition, since we still don't know all the nutrient requirements of the body, a varied diet will help increase your odds of getting all the nutrients your body may need.

Rule 4. Limit fat.

Avoid gravies, breading, and rich sauces. Eat less meat and more fish and poultry. Cut fat off of meat before cooking. Bake, broil, steam, roast, or stew rather than frying. Also, watch for hidden fats: It isn't just the sugar that is bad in cakes, cookies, doughnuts, ice cream, and chocolate candies—it's also the fat.

But don't decide never to eat fatty foods. Your body needs a certain amount of fat and cholesterol. People sometimes eliminate fat to such an extreme degree that they have menstrual and sexual problems because their bodies have no fats to produce needed hormones. Fats also help to retard hunger pangs and make you feel satisfied, and they are necessary for proper absorption of the fat-soluble vitamins.

You don't have to give up eggs completely, either. Even if you have a high cholesterol level, the latest medical advice is that you can have two or three eggs per week. If your cholesterol level is normal, you can eat more.

Rule 5. Limit use of alcohol and caffeine.

We have already discussed the insomnia-producing effects of alcohol and caffeine, so you know that cutting them down drastically is one of the most important things you can do to improve your sleep.

If you miss having something to drink at night, try sparkling mineral water or herbal tea instead of an alcoholic drink. Or drink seltzer (carbonated water), plain water, or club soda with a twist of lemon or lime. During the day, drink six to eight glasses of water instead of caffeine or alcohol drinks.

When You Eat Can Affect Your Sleep

It might seem logical to have a large, heavy dinner late in the evening, since a heavy meal tends to make you drowsy—but it also makes your digestive system work hard, which can keep you awake during the night. So don't eat a large, heavy meal shortly before bedtime—it's an invitation to a bad night's sleep.

Instead, to ensure sound sleep, eat a large breakfast, a moderate lunch, and a light dinner—and don't eat heavy, rich foods before bedtime. (This also can help you lose weight, since the latest research shows that calories consumed early in the day are used up more efficiently by the body.)

So make your evening meal a light one, and be sure that it contains some protein such as fish, chicken, or a vegetable protein. The protein will help prevent hunger pangs in the night.

Some nutritionists are even more precise in their instructions: If you have trouble falling asleep, you should eat a dinner that includes a protein, carbohydrate, and fat, about four hours before bedtime, and a snack of whole-grain carbohydrate, about two hours before bedtime. If you tend to awaken in the middle of the night, they say, move the dinner up to about two hours before bedtime and eat the snack at bedtime. We have had no experience with this diet, but we suggest that you might test it out for yourself and do whatever works best for you.

What Not to Eat

Stay away from snacks that are likely to give you indigestion or heart-burn, such as fatty foods, heavily garlic-flavored food, or highly spiced foods. If gas disturbs your sleep, avoid beans, cucumbers, or other foods that you have found cause you to have gas.

Many people are sensitive to monosodium glutamate (MSG). MSG can cause many symptoms, including insomnia. If you notice that insomnia occurs on nights that you have eaten Chinese food, MSG may be your problem.

If You Are on a Weight-Loss Diet

People who are losing weight may sleep poorly and awaken frequently, especially in the second half of the night. Also, patients who have the severe weight loss of anorexia nervosa often find that their sleep improves when they start eating and gaining weight. We don't suggest that you stop dieting, but you might try a low-calorie bedtime snack to avoid nighttime awakenings.

Sometimes, thyroid function may affect both weight and sleep. Hyperthyroidism is associated with weight loss and short sleep, with excessive amounts of delta sleep. Hypothyroidism results in weight gain and long sleep.

Food-Allergy Insomnia

Food allergies may cause insomnia. Respiratory allergies can keep you awake, too, but you're more likely to be aware of such allergies, due to obvious symptoms such as sneezing and itchy eyes. You usually know it is due to something like ragweed, dust, mold, or cat dander. Food allergies are more subtle, and you might not think of them as a possible cause of your insomnia.

In infants, food allergies can cause colic or waking and crying in the middle of the night. In adults, food-allergy reactions can cause difficulty in getting to sleep or frequent awakenings.

In infants, milk often is the culprit. Dr. A. Kahn of the Pediatric Sleep Laboratory of the Free University of Brussels, Belgium, studied 33 infants who had insomnia and found that almost all of them had allergies to milk. Their sleep became normal after elimination of milk from their diets. Insomnia reappeared when, as a trial, they were given milk again.

Sometimes, a baby's colic can be improved by giving unheated milk instead of warmed milk. If this does not help, an allergy may be involved. Discuss with the baby's doctor whether breast milk or a nonmilk formula should be used.

You may need to meet with an allergist to discover what is causing an allergic reaction. In both children and adults, the foods that are most commonly associated with food allergy are milk, corn, wheat, chocolate, nuts, egg whites, seafood, red and yellow dyes, and yeast. Relatives of the suspected food also may cause problems: For example, if you are allergic to corn, you probably also will be allergic to foods that are related to corn—corn starch, sorbitol, mannitol, corn syrup, dextrose, caramel color, corn oil, and corn bran.

Removal of the suspected food from the diet often results in the immediate restoration of normal sleep. However, it may take a week or two, so give it time. If you want to prove that a particular food truly did cause your insomnia, reintroduce it back into your diet after several weeks and see if the sleep disturbances come back. Be your own sleep therapist and experiment.

Night-Eating Syndrome

This condition, sometimes called night-time hunger, nocturnal eating, or the "Dagwood syndrome," occurs when a person awakens in the middle of the night and can't go back to sleep without eating. Sometimes, the urge to raid the refrigerator is uncontrollable. The syndrome may be caused by certain medical conditions, such as ulcer; by not eating right during the day; or by dieting. In many cases, though, it is a conditioned desire for food. People, even infants, can get conditioned to expecting food in the middle of the night.

If you have this problem, first see your doctor to check out if there is a medical condition that can be treated. Otherwise, try to break yourself of the habit gradually, realizing that this probably is a conditioned hunger. Once you have broken the habit, you'll probably sleep as well without eating. Eating frequent small meals during the day or drinking a glass of water when you awaken during the night may help.

Another cause of night-eating syndrome may be hypoglycemia (low blood sugar). Though this condition is controversial, even the American Medical Association recognizes that it exists in some patients. When your blood sugar drops, you wake up hungry. A good solution is a protein snack before bedtime. The protein metabolizes slowly and helps to prevent a drop in your blood-sugar level. Don't eat snacks containing a lot of sugar, though: Sugar causes your blood-sugar level to rise rapidly and then plummet. Experiment, and check it out for yourself. You might want to get a five- or six-hour glucose-tolerance test to determine if you do have hypoglycemia.

Vitamins and Minerals That Can Help You Sleep

Nutritional deficiencies or poor absorption of nutrients can cause chronic insomnia. The B vitamins, calcium, magnesium, zinc, copper, and iron all have been shown to affect sleep.

Today, with so many of us eating on the run, often without easy access to fresh-from-the-farm foods, it makes sense to take vitamin-mineral supplements, particularly if you have any special problems such as a sleep disturbance.

In this section, we'll discuss the vitamins and minerals that affect sleep.

The B Vitamins

The B vitamins regulate the body's use of tryptophan and other amino acids, and so it is logical for them to be involved in sleep. (We'll talk more about tryptophan later.) The vital B-complex vitamins are used up by cigarette smoking, alcohol, and stress, and may be especially lacking in women who are on birth-control pills.

Several studies have been done on various B vitamins and sleep. For example, supplements of vitamin B3 (also called niacin or niacinamide) often help people who have depression along with insomnia. Sometimes, 50 to 100 mg of niacin per day can improve mild depression, as well as the accompanying insomnia. Niacin also has been found to increase the effectiveness of tryptophan in promoting sleep. Studies by Dr. Connie Robinson at the University of Alabama Department of Neurosciences show that niacin prolongs REM sleep and decreases the awake time of insomniac patients. It is reported to be particularly helpful for patients who fall asleep readily but who can't return to sleep after awakening during the night. Niacin may cause flushing, but this is a natural reaction and should not be a cause for concern.

Vitamin B12 also can be helpful. In 1983, a study in which vitamin B12 restored normal sleep in an insomniac who had difficulty in falling asleep and had frequent awakenings was reported in the journal *Sleep* by three scientists from the National Institute of Mental Health. Drs. Behrooz Kamgar-Parsi, Thomas Wehr, and J. Christian Gillin reported that the patient was able to maintain normal sleep-wake cycles for the first time in ten years after taking B12 supplements.

Another part of the vitamin-B family—folic acid—can be helpful in some cases of insomnia. Dr. J. S. Howard III reported in the journal *Psychosomatics* that insomnia can be a side effect of folic-acid deficiency; such insomnias can be treated with 2 to 5 mg of folic acid per day.

Other relatives in the vitamin-B family—inositol and pantothenic acid—also have been found to be helpful in some patients when taken an hour or two before bedtime.

However, in some people, the B vitamins can act as energizers and cause overstimulation and sleeplessness. Idiosyncrasies like this are one of the reasons you should work with a professional person whenever possible when taking supplements, especially in large amounts.

Calcium

It is well known that calcium has a calming effect on the central nervous system and is essential for normal sleep. A 1978 study at the University of Alabama showed that even a minor calcium deficiency can lead to muscle tension and insomnia.

Calcium is one of the most important minerals of the nervous system. Calcium and its partner, magnesium, act as natural relaxants. Conversely, they are rapidly depleted under stressful conditions.

The ability to absorb calcium often decreases with age, so insomnia in people over age 50 sometimes can be a result of poor calcium absorption. This condition often coexists with the progressive bone loss of osteoporosis.

The calcium requirement currently recommended by experts in the field (the recommendations change often) is 800 mg for adult men and women and 1,200 mg for teenagers and pregnant women, lactating women, and women after menopause. But it is difficult for most people to get the recommended amounts: Many adults have decreased or eliminated their milk consumption because of allergies or lactose intolerance, and many others simply do not like milk. For these people, it is a good idea to take a calcium supplement. Take it just before bedtime. Calcium supplements also should contain magnesium and potassium to aid absorption and create the proper balance with other minerals.

Magnesium

Magnesium is a natural sedative; it is soothing and helps guard against anxiety. Some insomniacs have been shown to suffer from a magnesium deficiency. Several clinicians say that for such people, 250 to 300 mg of magnesium taken daily usually can correct the magnesium deficiency and produce sound sleep.

In one study, involving more than 200 insomnia patients, Drs. W. Davis and F. Ziady of the University of Pretoria (South Africa) reported that many patients given magnesium supplements were helped. They fell asleep more quickly, had uninterrupted sleep, and awakened refreshed. They also found that anxiety and tension levels were diminished during the day.

Magnesium also is being found helpful (along with potassium) in people who complain of constant fatigue. One study published in *Current Therapeutic Research* showed that 87 of 100 persons complaining of constant fatigue experienced increased energy and strength within five to ten days after beginning magnesium and potassium supplements. In another study published in the *Journal of Abdominal Surgery*, 75 of 80 subjects said that their tiredness and weakness diminished within three days to two weeks after beginning magnesium and potassium supplements. They said that they slept better and awakened without their usual morning exhaustion.

When magnesium is taken, it should be in balanced proportions of two parts calcium to one part magnesium.

Zinc

People suffering from insomnia may be deficient in zinc. Occasionally, this deficiency has been linked to frequent nighttime waking and crying in infants. You might try taking zinc supplements for a few weeks to see if your sleep problem improves. But zinc supplements should be given to infants and children only by prescription from a nutritionally oriented pediatrician. Read the label on your child's vitamin bottle; if zinc is not included in the supplement and if your child awakens frequently during the night, you may want to discuss with the pediatrician whether to use a child's vitamin formula that includes calcium, magnesium, and zinc.

Copper and Iron

Poor sleep can occur from too little copper or iron in the diet, according to a U.S. Department of Agriculture (USDA) psychologist. In 1988, Dr. James G. Penland of the USDA Agricultural Research Service reported on a series of five carefully controlled, long term studies of trace-element nutrition and sleep. He asked women eight questions each morning about how long and how well they slept the night before. Their responses were later correlated with dietary intake and blood-plasma levels of the element in question.

Of the seven elements studied, copper, iron, and aluminum most strongly altered sleep patterns. Reducing the daily intake of copper or iron "increased sleep time and decreased its quality," he said. High doses of aluminum—a nonessential element found in many antacids—reduced sleep quality. He said that regular antacid users "can easily get 1,000 milligrams of aluminum a day"—the amount used in the study.

In another USDA study at the Human Nutrition Research Center in Grand Forks, North Dakota, a diet with low levels of iron and copper was fed to volunteers. For three months, a group of women was given meals containing less than a third of the USDA's recommended daily allowance (RDA) of copper. A second group received less than a third of the RDA of iron. Both groups also were studied for three months on normal diets.

When deprived of normal amounts of either copper or iron, the women reported that they slept poorly, although in different ways. Those getting insufficient copper found that they slept longer, yet felt worse when they awoke, compared to their sleep when not on a copper-deficient diet. Those getting too little iron also slept longer, but woke more often during the night.

Researchers have known for years that copper and iron affect brain activity. Copper is involved in making norepinephrine, a brain chemical responsible for the brain's general arousal. Iron is essential for making dopamine, a chemical found in areas of the brain involved in motor activities, as well as for making hemoglobin, which supplies oxygen to the body and brain through the bloodstream. Thus, it is not surprising that different levels of copper and iron could affect sleep.

Copper or iron supplements should be taken *only* under the guidance of a professional person knowledgeable in nutrition. Too much of either copper or iron can cause serious side effects, and both minerals need to be in careful balance with other minerals in the body. In men, especially, iron overload can be a problem, with the excess iron conflicting with the absorption of zinc and being deposited in some of the soft tissues of the body.

Keeping Track

Most of us aren't used to thinking in terms of vitamin and mineral balance, but if you haven't been helped sufficiently from the changes you've made so far with the program, you might want to explore these vitamins and minerals for yourself. Keep a Sleep Log as you try the vitamin and mineral supplements and other nutritional changes. If you think you have found something useful, double check by going off it again for a week or two, then reinstate it and see if you still get the good results.

Tryptophan

As this book goes to press, there is a great deal of controversy about tryptophan. Tryptophan is not a drug, but a naturally occurring amino acid that is essential in helping the body build protein. It is found in a variety of foods, including milk, meat, fish, poultry, eggs, beans, peanuts, cheese, and leafy green vegetables, and you can buy it as a supplement. Many sleep researchers, including those at the leading sleep disorders centers, have recommended taking tryptophan in the evening to treat poor sleep.

Tryptophan is important for sleep because it is the raw material out of which the brain manufactures the neurotransmitter chemical serotonin. One of the functions of serotonin is to slow down nerve activity, therefore inducing sleep.

Now, suddenly we are finding that some people who have been taking tryptophan over long periods are developing a strange set of symptoms: aching muscles and joints, sometimes fatigue and fever or skin rash, and sometimes an elevated number of white blood cells known as eosinophils. The condition has been named eosinophilia-myalgia syndrome.

We don't yet know the reason, so we can only speculate: Could it be that just a few people react adversely to tryptophan, much the same as the small number of people who have adverse side-effects to aspirin? Nearly all tryptophan comes from Japan—could tryptophan somehow have been tainted either at the source or in the manufacture of tablets by a distributor? Is there some other factor, as some people experience these symptoms, yet have not taken tryptophan? Does it only occur when tryptophan is taken in combination with other medications or certain foods? Is long term use the determining factor?

The first case of the strange symptoms was reported in 1988 by Dr. Joseph Duffy of Mayo Clinic. In 1989 a physician in Albuquerque, New Mexico, who had a female patient with similar symptoms remembered the report and referred the woman to Mayo Clinic. Within a few days other cases began to show up in New Mexico. As doctors began discussing the symptoms with their colleagues, they realized there were other probable cases. Within days, state departments of health began compiling the data, and continue to track it now.

Our present recommendation—and the U.S. government's—is simply to stop taking tryptophan until we learn all the facts. If you have any of the symptoms described and don't know the cause, contact your doctor.

We cannot predict the outcome of the current investigation, but we can tell you about people's past experience with tryptophan. At first there were many different opinions expressed in scientific literature as to the effectiveness of tryptophan. A lot of disagreement arose from the fact that doses studied in early research were typically too low to have any consistent effect. In addition, these studies were performed on good sleepers, not on insomniacs, so there was no apparent effectiveness. Later experiments used higher dosages and insomniacs as test subjects.

Currently there are at least 25 studies suggesting that taking tryptophan in the evening helps about half of all insomniacs, both those who have difficulties falling asleep and those who awaken often during the night. For example, Dr. Ernest Hartmann, director of the Sleep Disorders Center of Newton-Wellesley Hospital in Boston, and his colleagues gave each of ten men with mild insomnia doses of tryptophan on different nights, as well as a dummy placebo. With the placebos, the men needed an average of about 24 minutes to fall asleep, but with tryptophan they needed only about 12 minutes. Later, the researchers lowered dosages and found that doses as low as 1 gram were effective in many, but they found 2 grams to have the best effect.

Dr. Gila Lindsley and her colleagues, working in Dr. Hartmann's clinic, compared the effectiveness of 1 gram of tryptophan with 100 milligrams of Seconal and 30 milligrams of Dalmane, two of the more potent prescription sleeping pills available. Their test subjects comprised 54 serious insomniacs who either woke up often in the middle of the night or dozed half awake most of the night. In these patients 1 gram of tryptophan was as effective as either of the two prescription drugs.

A study by Dr. Dietrich Schneider-Helmert, of the University of Amsterdam in the Netherlands, suggests that you don't have to take tryptophan every night, since its effectiveness is cumulative, and in fact, works best after several days. When you are having poor sleep, he has suggested that you take tryptophan on three consecutive nights, say Monday, Tuesday, and Wednesday nights, then not take any for the next four nights. Contrary to the effects of typical sleeping pills, the four nights without tryptophan often were at least as good, if not better, than the three nights on tryptophan. This schedule was repeated in chronic insomniacs for at least three months until their sleep was normalized. "It re-established normal sleep functions in the large majority of severe and chronic insomniacs," Schneider-Helmert reported.)

Tryptophan is typically bought in health-food stores in 500 mg. tablets. (The label may say l-tryptophan, which is the form used clinically.

Both what you eat and don't eat with tryptophan is important. When animal proteins such as meat, fish, eggs, or dairy foods are eaten at the same time as you take tryptophan, the rise in blood tryptophan that is caused by taking the tryptophan tablets does not necessarily cause a corresponding rise in brain tryptophan. This is because it is very difficult for any amino acid from the blood to get into the brain. If certain other amino acids are floating around in your bloodstream, they use up part of the transport system that goes from the blood into the brain and that keeps the tryptophan from getting through. Thus, all the ingested tryptophan is probably circulating in your bloodstream, but not getting into your brain in adequate amounts. Therefore, it has been recommended that you not take tryptophan with protein.

It takes about an hour for tryptophan to enter your brain and be changed into serotonin, the chemical that insomniacs want to increase. So, for best results, it has been recommended that you have dinner at least four hours before going to bed, and that you take the tryptophan one hour before bed.

Some researchers have recommended combining tryptophan with 250 milligrams of niacinamide (vitamin B3) and a slice of whole-wheat bread spread with avocado or some other carbohydrate food. This combination apparently makes tryptophan's sleep-producing effect last further into the night. It also has been recommended that insomniacs try taking tryptophan with fruit juice. (The carbohydrate in fruit juice seems to help transport tryptophan into the brain.)

Tryptophan needs the chemical pyridoxal-5-phosphate to be converted into serotonin. P5P is made by the body from pyridoxine (vitamin B6). Some people lack the enzyme that converts vitamin B6 to P5P, which may be a reason why some people do not respond to tryptophan therapy. One patient with insomnia, the president of a medical company, said he had a blood test for amino acids that showed low tryptophan and P5P. By taking both tryptophan and P5P an hour before bedtime, his sleeping pattern improved greatly.

An amino acid fractionation test, as well as vitamin and mineral assessments, may be tests of the future for insomniacs at sleep centers.

· · · ● ● ● · ·

Until the investigation of eosinophilia-myalgia syndrome is completed, do not use tryptophan. If you have been using tryptophan, check with your physician; then if you have a sleep problem, ask for his or her recommendation on what to do.

If the time ever comes when the ban is lifted and tryptophan is shown to be safe and you want to see if it improves your sleep, start with two grams, taking it with fruit juice about three hours after your evening meal (about one hour before bedtime) for three consecutive nights. Do not eat cheese and crackers or milk as a bedtime snack if you take tryptophan since they contain other amino acids besides tryptophan. If two grams are not effective, you may take up to four grams. If two grams are effective, try decreasing that dose to one gram (two tablets) or even 500 mg (one tablet) to see if you can get by on less.

· · · ● ● ● · ·

Herbal Remedies

The best teas for inducing sleep, say herbalists, are those made with chamomile, valerian, primrose, catnip, almonds, fennel, melissa, passion flower, rosemary, skullcap, or hops. Early American settlers used bergamot tea, pennyroyal, and lemon balm. Gentian root has been used for hundreds of years as a sleeping aid and relaxant in Europe. The Hopi use sand verbena.

Dr. Peter Leathwood of Nestle Research Laboratories in Switzerland studied the aqueous extract of valerian root. He reported in the journal *Pharmacology, Biochemistry and Behavior* that in a controlled study with 128 people, freshly prepared valerian did improve sleep quality, and there was no morning-after hangover effect. Subjects also took less time to go to sleep, especially people who normally had poor sleep. However, a commercial preparation of valerian did not have these effects. Valerian seldom is used in the United States and Britain, but is popular for its sedative properties in France, Germany, and Switzerland.

We have no personal experience with the use of herbal preparations. If you decide to try any of them, we suggest that you work with someone who is an expert in herbs, since overdoses of herbs or the wrong combinations, as with any substance, can cause side effects. Health-food stores and other outlets usually carry herbal combinations for insomnia. Try a low dosage first, and don't overdo it.

···· 10 ····

Make Exercise Work for Your Sleep

There's a story that doctors like to tell: A man was depressed, couldn't sleep, was failing at work, and felt so bad that he decided to commit suicide by running himself to death so his family could collect the insurance. So he went out and ran as long as he could. But he didn't die, so he decided to try again the next day and ran faster and farther. He kept running for six weeks, and then he felt so good that he decided to live.

Exercise can make you feel good and sleep well. It doesn't always work (there are insomniac athletes, including some Olympic stars, so there's no guarantee that exercise will help you sleep). But it can be one of the most important things you do to turn insomnia into sound sleep.

As part of your total insomnia program, be sure to include exercise. You must tire your body if you hope to sleep well. Fitness definitely facilitates good sleep. This has been shown in the laboratory at the Royal Edinburgh Hospital in Scotland, where army recruits who worked out on a treadmill to increase fitness took less time to go to sleep and had fewer awakenings.

Often, people who complain of insomnia are sedentary and rarely exercise. Regular exercise not only helps you go to sleep more easily, but also deepens sleep. Athletes and other physically fit people show more delta sleep than do nonathletes.

However, exercise during any one day may or may not deepen sleep that night, depending on the time of day when the exercise was performed. Exercise in the morning or during the late evening has less effect than exercise in the late afternoon or early evening.

You don't have to exercise to exhaustion, but you should engage in some physical activity to the point where your pulse is elevated on a regular, planned basis. This not only will help your sleep, but also will provide several side benefits. It burns calories, increases circulation, improves the heart and lungs, builds stronger bones to help ward off osteoporosis, tones muscles, reduces cholesterol levels, and lowers blood pressure. All these things will make you look and feel better.

Another reason you'll feel better is because exercise produces mood elevators called *endorphins*, which are naturally occurring brain chemicals that relieve depression and produce a sense of well-being. One 34-year-old patient had a severe case of insomnia that appeared to be due to a combination of anxiety and depression. Before he was treated with long term psychotherapy or drugs, he was urged to take up some regular exercise. He chose running and, after several weeks of daily running, he had such a powerful feeling of well-being that his anxiety and depression lifted and his insomnia totally disappeared.

The Temperature Connection

The benefit of exercise in combating insomnia has been well known for a long time, but sleep researchers recently have come up with some fascinating new information. They have learned that it's not just the exercise itself that's beneficial, but the increase in body temperature.

It works like this: In general, if you are a daytime worker, the temperature of your body goes up during the day and down during the night, usually peaking at midafternoon and bottoming out around 4 or 5 A.M. The body-temperature peaks are about 2 degrees Fahrenheit higher than the troughs when you are young, less as you grow older. We don't know why this happens, but it seems to be a built-in biological rhythm that all of us have. In insomniacs, the temperature rhythm is much flatter and shallower than in normal sleepers. Their temperature increases less during the day, since they are less alert and less active; their temperature doesn't decrease as much during the night, and their sleep is shallow and fragmented.

If you can increase your body temperature about five or six hours before going to bed, the temperature then will drop most as you are ready to go to sleep. The trough deepens, and sleep becomes deeper, with fewer awakenings.

We now think that exercise helps sleep because it causes this increase in body temperature. So if you play tennis and are tired a few hours later, it may be not just that you are tired from the exertion, but that you become sleepy from the drop in your body temperature.

Any exercise is good if it is intensive enough to raise the core (inside) body temperature about 2 degrees Fahrenheit for about 20 minutes. The type of exercise you do will depend on your interests and your level of fitness. Try different types of exercise and see what it does to your sleep.

This temperature theory also can explain the sleep-producing effects of a hot tub, and you may be able to use this phenomenon to trick the system. On days that you don't have time to exercise, try this: Late in the afternoon or early evening, raise the body temperature by sitting in a hot tub or bathtub filled with hot water for 20 minutes. The bath has to be hot, not just comfortable, and if it is a bathtub, you have to keep running the hot water to *keep* it hot. A hot shower will work only if you are willing to stay in the shower for a full 20 minutes. You can try it and see what it does to your sleep, and at what time of afternoon or evening it works best for you.

The Activity Connection

It may sound strange, but many insomniacs who come into our insomnia program seem "frozen." They never seem to relax, and they never seem to stretch themselves, mentally or physically. They appear to be afraid that they won't have the strength to do things or will be worn out. We often have to teach them to push themselves—to work hard, to play hard, and to learn the joys both of exercise and of complete relaxation. These kinds of highs and lows seem to improve sleep more than if a person stays frozen at the same level all the time.

Now research has been reported that shows why this is so. Dr. Charles Pollak, of New York Hospital-Cornell Medical Center, found that people with insomnia have the same flatness in their activity during the day-night cycle as they do in their temperature fluctuations. They have less body movement in the daytime and more body movement at night. This is not the only factor, of course, but it is one factor to consider. Try to be as active as you can in the daytime and don't let yourself "freeze" into a pattern of boredom and routine.

Effective Exercise

The favorite exercise for patients in our program is brisk walking. Sometimes, just a walk a day can keep insomnia away. Walk briskly—arms swinging—hard enough to get your heart rate up, get you breathing hard, and get your activity level and core temperature up. Within minutes, walking starts to reduce tension and anxiety.

If you like to bicycle, that's good, too. If you use a stationary one, you can even do it while watching TV or reading. The important thing is to find something you enjoy. If it's fun, you won't skip it—you'll keep doing it.

You can get your activity- and temperature-raising exercise with running, swimming, bicycling, walking, dancing, skating, tennis, skiing, or doing aerobic workouts. Or you can choose more than one and alternate on different days. (Just working around the house or garden does not count unless you do something strenuous, such as vacuuming or raking leaves, that raises body temperature and heart rate.)

Remember, the more you do, the more you'll be able to do. If you don't feel well on a given day, then feel free to skip that day. Exercise again the next day. But don't go off your exercise program for very long, because fitness starts to deteriorate after only 72 hours, and there's a chance your sleep problems may come back. It's been shown that regular exercisers who skip their customary exercise get less deep sleep that night than usual.

What if you feel too tired to exercise? Don't put off exercising until some nebulous future when you might have more energy. Contrary to what most people think, moderate exercising when you are tired can actually perk you up and make you feel better. It also helps to counteract chronic fatigue. If you are too tired to go out or if you are insecure about your looks or skills, work with an exercise class on TV or buy an exercise video cassette.

You need to get yourself onto an exercise program even if you think that you're too fatigued to lift a finger. Most insomniacs think that they need to sleep better first, and then they will be able to exercise. It is the other way around: You have to exercise first, and then you will sleep better.

Caution: When people begin exercise programs, they often do too much too fast, which can result in muscle aches and pains. Avoid overexertion. Check with your doctor, plan a schedule to suit your own fitness level, and gradually increase your activity level over the weeks. At any time, if your pulse pounds or becomes irregular or you feel worse after your exercise periods, immediately stop exercising and contact your physician before resuming.

Your doctor also may want to follow what the exercise does to any problem you have. For instance, if you have diabetes or high blood pressure, the exercise may prove to be so beneficial that you may need to have the dosages of your medications lowered!

You should see your doctor before you begin your exercise program and get specific recommendations, especially if:

- You are overweight
- You are over 45 years old and not accustomed to regular exercise
- You have any kind of heart trouble or have had a heart attack
- Your doctor has said that your blood pressure is too high and not under control, or you don't know whether your blood pressure is normal
- You frequently have pain or pressure in the chest, neck, shoulder, or arm after you exercise
- You experience extreme breathlessness after mild exertion
- You have bone or joint problems
- You have a family history of early heart trouble
- You often feel faint or dizzy
- You have a medical condition that might need special attention, such as diabetes

Other Guidelines

It is not necessary to exercise every day. The usual recommendation is to exercise three times per week (including 5 to 10 minutes of warm-up, 20 minutes in the aerobic range (when your heart rate is elevated), then a slowdown and a shower).

During the warm-up, do light, slow, nonstressful exercise. Simply move your joints through their full range of motion. Lift your arms, make circles, stretch your legs, stand on your tiptoes. Or simply do the same exercise you plan to do, but do it slowly and less vigorously. Warm-ups raise your body temperature, make muscles more pliant, and increase blood flow to make more oxygen available for energy production. Stretches, also important, help to prevent muscle and ligament strains from any strenuous exertion. During your warm-up and stretching, avoid forceful or wrenching movements and concentrate on loosening and relaxing your muscles, easing into the exercise slowly.

Then, if you are fit, do at least 20 minutes of your chosen exercise strenuously enough to achieve your temperature increase. If you are unfit, you may first have to be satisfied with less than 20 minutes at peak exertion–say, 5 minutes. Then gradually work up to 20 minutes.

Finally, allow at least a five-minute cool-down period of about the same intensity as your warm-up exercise—walking around for awhile will do it.

Although sleep researchers suggest that we need a 2-degree-Fahrenheit increase in our core body temperature, it is hard to picture a person jogging, then stopping periodically to measure core temperature, which needs to be done rectally. You can use the heart rate "target zone" as a guide. Here's how it works: Take 220 minus your age. This gives your maximum heart rate for a given age. From that number, compute 60 percent and 75 percent—between them is your "target zone." During the aerobic part of your exercise, strive to have your heart rate in your target range. (Take your pulse for ten seconds and multiply by six to get your heart rate.)

You also can use the chart on page 135 to find your target zone.

If you don't want to do all this measuring, you can exercise until you are slightly breathless but still able to talk; exercise experts say this usually is just about at your aerobic threshold.

Below your target range, you are not exercising enough. Above it, you could be doing more damage than good. Again, you need to build up your tolerance. In the beginning, if you are totally out of shape, you probably should spend no more than a few minutes in this target range. Gradually, you build up your time, first to 10, then 15, then 20 minutes—plus your warm-up and cool-down times. After six months or more of regular exercise, you can exercise at up to 85 percent of your maximum heart rate if you wish.

You should discontinue any exercise and rest if you have tightness or pain in the chest, dizziness, severe breathlessness, nausea, abnormal

YOUR AEROBIC HEART RATE TARGET ZONE

Age, years	Target zone, beats/minute	Maximum heart rate, beats/minute
20	120–150	200
25	117–146	195
30	114–142	190
35	111–138	185
40	108–135	180
45	105–131	175
50	102–127	170
55	99–123	165
60	96–120	160
65	93–116	155
70	90–113	150

To find your target zone, look for the age category closest to your age and read the line across. For example, if you are 30, your target zone is 114 to 142 beats per minute. If you are 43, the closest age on the chart is 45; the target zone is 105 to 131 beats per minute.

Courtesy American Heart Association. Reprinted with permission.

heart rate, profuse sweating, or sudden flu-like symptoms. If these symptoms persist, consult a physician.

How Soon Will You See Results?

Within two to three weeks of beginning your exercise program, you should start to see some results in the way you feel. You'll probably have more energy and be less tense during the day and evening—and you'll likely be sleeping better.

Keep the program up and you may never want to quit because you'll feel so good.

···· 11 ····

Resetting Your Sleep Clock

In 1938, Dr. Nathaniel Kleitman of the University of Chicago and his assistant, Dr. Bruce H. Richardson, isolated themselves in the clammy depths of Mammoth Cave, Kentucky, to see what would happen to a person living in an environment without a daily rhythm of light and darkness. They lived underground for 33 days in a constant, foggy chill of 54 degrees Fahrenheit, without any idea of what time it was. The scientists lived an artifical routine of 19 hours awake and 9 hours asleep and studied correlations of body temperature and other factors.

In 1962, a young French geologist, Michel Siffre, also studied life without any time clues. In the Alps, at an altitude of 7,500 feet, he found a cave that descended vertically for 90 feet, snaked around in an S-shaped tunnel, then dropped farther underground to about 400 feet. The cave was totally dark, the floor solid ice, the temperature icy cold. He stayed there alone for two months, his only contact by telephone with two friends at the surface. He called to tell them when he went to bed, when he woke up, and when he ate a meal. He kept a diary of his activities and a chart of the time and date he thought it was, while his friends kept a corresponding chart of the actual time and date.

Most time-free research today is not so rugged. Subjects usually live in soundproof apartments with the windows bricked up and the clocks removed. The apartments usually contain a bed, an exercise station, a work station, a kitchen, a stereo, and a VCR, but no TV or radio that would give subjects the time. The volunteers can work, eat, and sleep whenever they want. They sometimes have occasional contact with outsiders, but only with technicians who are carefully trained not to give any hint of which day or night it might be. For example, every time a male technician goes into the apartment, he has to shave first so that the patients cannot tell from his "five o'clock shadow" what time it is. Meals are served on demand. Core temperature, hormone levels, and other vital functions usually are monitored and computer analyzed, along with psychological and behavioral changes. The volunteers are observed from the outside by video cameras and, when they are sleeping, their brain waves are recorded.

But caves still give the most insulation from noise and the most complete sense of isolation, so in 1989 there was a new cave-dweller: Stefania Follini. She climbed 30 feet underground into a cave near Carlsbad, New Mexico, for a 131-day experiment. She lived in a tiny Plexiglas house in the cave and, for entertainment, had a computer and some 400 books. Part of the research was geared to exploring how humans might react during long, lonely interplanetary space-flights.

Unfailingly, in all these experiments, people cut loose from society's synchronization, and their built-in rhythms begin to "free-run" into their own sleep-wake cycles, often producing a day much longer than 24 hours. Follini, for example, fell into a routine of staying awake about 23 hours, then sleeping for 10; later, she was awake for even longer. Other people in the time-free environments have had sleep-wake rhythms that ran anywhere from 26 to 30 hours.

An Upset in Rhythm May be Causing Your Insomnia

Our rhythms of about 24 hours are called *circadian,* from the Latin *circa,* meaning about, and *dian,* meaning a day. Because they are integral to our sleeping and waking, and because they can get out of whack, they can be a major factor in insomnia.

If you can sleep well, but not at a time when you want to sleep or when you feel you should, you may have a circadian-rhythm disorder. For example, some people sleep well from 6 A.M. to 2 P.M. or from 7 P.M. to 2 A.M., but can't sleep from 11 P.M. to 7 A.M. when they want to. In rare cases, the insomnia caused by a rhythm disorder shows itself periodically, say two weeks of poor sleep every five weeks or so. If you think this might be a possibility, keep your Sleep Log for at least two months to determine if there is a rhythmic cycle to your insomnia.

Different People Have Different Rhythms

Researchers have found that the lengths of our sleep-wake rhythms change during our lifetimes. Newborns do not have a circadian rhythm, but develop one within the first few months of life. From about 6 months to about 14 years, the rhythm is very close to 24 hours. Most children get up easily most mornings at about the same time and fall asleep at about the same time each night.

Then, somewhere during the teen years, the rhythm slows down, so that the internal clock is always slower than the clock on the wall. That's why adolescents don't want to go to sleep when the clock says it's 11 P.M. Their bodys' clocks say it couldn't be more than 8 P.M. Adolescents also have a hard time getting up to go to school. When the clock on the wall says 7 A.M., their bodies probably say it couldn't be more than about 4 A.M. For at least ten years, most adolescents have to contend with an internal clock that runs slowly, at around 26 to 30 hours. The only way to squeeze this slow internal clock into the world's 24-hour schedule is to get up in the morning earlier than the body says it is time to get up. It isn't easy—in fact, it's a constant, biologically imposed struggle in most adolescents and young adults to get up in the morning. It is not that the younger generation is bad, lazy, or shiftless—their clocks simply are running on a slower time.

Luckily, in the late 20s or early 30s, the internal clock typically speeds up again, so that most of the rest of our lives we are living more comfortably on this 24-hour planet.

However, as we grow older, the internal clock usually (but not always) speeds up further. It then may become shorter than 24 hours. That's why Grandma typically goes to bed so early, say at 7 or 8 in the evening—because her body says it's midnight. The same Grandma wakes up by 2 or 3 A.M., because her body clock, being fast, says it's morning.

Another thing that happens in old age is that the rhythm becomes much flatter. While the young adult typically shows a change of about 2 degrees Fahrenheit in core body temperature between day and night, you can consider yourself lucky as a 75-year-old if the difference between night and day is 1/2 degree. Other sleep characteristics flatten out, too. This is why, when we are younger and have strong circadian cycles, we are either quite clearly awake or quite clearly asleep. We have one period, during the night, when we sleep and one period, during the day, when we are awake. As we get older and our rhythms flatten, we usually are much closer to dozing day and night, taking naps during the day and being awake much more often at night. We don't need to sleep any longer or any shorter than when we were younger, but we spread our sleep and our wakefulness more evenly over the 24 hours.

The actual situation is even more complicated. At all ages, it appears that there's not one, but two clocks in our bodies. Researchers have pinpointed one as a neurological clock located in the brain as a nucleus of nerve cells close to where the optic nerves come together, so that the clock can be influenced by light. The other clock seems more like a buildup and decay of some chemical that gets used up during the day and then is replenished when we sleep. Different body functions are governed by the two clocks. Our temperature rhythm seems to be run by the neurological clock (as well as by the environment); our sleep-wake behavior and many other things are run by the buildup and decay clock. The problem is that these two clocks don't run exactly on the same schedule.

In the young adult, the neurological clock typically runs at about 25 hours, the buildup and decay clock at about 28 hours. Imagine having two bedroom clocks, one slowed to about 25 hours, the other slowed to about 28 hours. If you let these two clocks run for a week or two, you wouldn't have the foggiest idea what time it was. If you were stuck with such clocks, you would have to reset them every morning; for the rest of the day, you could pretty much tell what time it was. But by the next morning, they would already be a few hours apart and you would have to reset them again. That is exactly what we have to do with our bodies. To keep our two clocks close enough so that our bodies can function as a unit and we can be synchronized with the rest of the world, we have to reset the clocks once every 24 hours. The signal to reset the clocks is called a *zeitgeber*, a time-giver.

The best time-giver for the young is a regular wake-up time. It doesn't matter what time it is, but it should be regular. Young people have to reset their clocks by getting up early.

The best time-giver for the elderly is a regular bedtime. Older people have to stretch the clock by going to bed at a later time than they feel comfortable, so that they don't wake up the next morning at 3. (Of course, it doesn't really matter whether you wake up at 2 or 3 in the morning, as long as you're not concerned about it.)

The two ways to reset your clocks are by light and by activity. When your body wants to sleep at a time you want to be up, going out into sunlight and moving around can give you a very powerful stimulus that resets the clocks. Or you might expose yourself to very bright indoor lights at such times.

How You Might Be Upsetting Your Rhythm

Although circadian rhythms come from within our own bodies, our lifestyles can mess them up. If we don't give a strong zeitgeber to our body every morning or every evening, but sleep and wake in a random way whenever we feel like it, not only can the two internal clocks desynchronize, but we eventually can lose most aspects of rhythmicity. Then we are able to sleep or to wake only in very short episodes of one-half to three hours, day and night, just like a newborn baby. We no longer have a regular rhythm at all.

Usually, the disorganization starts with a few nights of insomnia. Not having slept well, you sleep late the next morning and then have trouble falling asleep the next night; then you sleep late again the next morning. Soon, your entire sleep system has moved up to a later time. It becomes almost impossible to fall asleep at the time you previously did.

Or if you take a nap the next day, you probably will be unable to sleep soundly the next night. A vicious circle develops and, gradually, sleep and wakefulness get spread almost evenly over the 24 hours. The circadian rhythm is lost. The situation can become so severe that you may lie in bed most of the day, and this weakens sleep even further. To avoid this problem: Always get up in the morning at the same time.

Tom Mustopheles, a 25-year-old mechanic, had been hit by a train, was hospitalized for three months, made a dramatic recovery, and seemed to be relatively normal except for a slight speech deficit and some problems with memory. His lawyers, however, advised him not to work until his damage suit was settled.

Tom had always been a loner, and he spent the next two years in a small apartment, reading, watching TV, and doing very little else. Whenever he needed food, he would get it from a nearby 24-hour grocery store. There were almost no zeitgebers in his environment. After about two months on this nonschedule, his sleep deteriorated and he felt increasingly tired. Gradually, he spent most of his time simply lying in bed—dozing, but never really sleeping. He also became quite weak.

After two years, while his lawsuit dragged on, Tom was referred to the insomnia clinic. Twenty-four-hour recordings revealed that he took frequent short naps throughout the day and night, rarely sleeping more than 30 minutes and rarely being alert more than an hour at a time. His body temperature showed no discernible circadian rhythm, only wide and random fluctuations.

Tom was urged to reestablish a regular day-night rhythm, but wasn't able to do it because he always felt tired. Finally, he hired a friend to keep him awake and active during the day, and he gradually narrowed his time in bed to the night. This had to be done slowly. In the beginning, he was up only from 11 A.M. to 2 P.M. Gradually, he extended that time by about one hour each week. Regular mealtimes and a slow increase in exercise during the middle of the day also were prescribed to reinforce the circadian rhythm. Over a period of six very difficult months, Tom reestablished a normal sleep-wake rhythm and felt better.

Then a settlement was reached in his lawsuit, and with the proceedings from it, Tom bought a small farm in New England. The very regular sleep-wake rhythm of a dairy farmer did wonders for him. He now manages the farm effectively, and his insomnia has totally disappeared.

If You're An Insomniac, You Need a Regular Rhythm

Rarely are things as dramatic as with Tom Mustopheles, but keeping your sleep schedule regular can work wonders. The more you suffer from insomnia, the more you need to maintain a regular sleep-wake rhythm, even if it's a struggle. This is why we recommend that even after a sleepless night, you drag yourself out of bed and try to be involved in physical activity throughout the day.

You must get up at the same time—no matter what. You may need to have your spouse drag you into the shower or set three alarm clocks and hide them around the room, but you must get up on time, the same time, every time.

If you usually can't fall asleep until 5 in the morning, try to force yourself to get up at, say, 8 in the morning. In a few days or weeks, you will get sleepier earlier at night, especially if you also use photo therapy (page 144) in the early morning hours.

Most of the time you can get a regular rhythm established on your own, but it doesn't always work. You may need to get professional help from a sleep disorders center.

Sunday Night Insomnia

One kind of disturbed rhythm that affects many people is "Sunday night insomnia." They have a terrible time sleeping Sunday night, and they and their family may think that they are lazy or don't want to face the work week, but it just as well may be a rearranged rhythm. Here's how it goes: On Friday night, Mary stayed up late because it wasn't a school or work night, and Saturday morning, she slept a few hours later than usual. Now her body clock is maybe two hours late. Saturday night she stayed up even later and Sunday morning slept even later, so her body clock is now four or more hours behind. If she tries to go to sleep at her regular bedtime on Sunday night, her body clock feels as if it were still early in the evening. No wonder she's not sleepy.

If Sunday night insomnia is a problem for you, then you should go to bed at a reasonable hour on Friday and Saturday nights and wake yourself up Saturday and Sunday morning at the regular time. Even if you don't go to bed at a reasonable hour, you still should wake yourself up at your regular time. You'll be a little tired, but you will not have messed up your clock and you'll be able to sleep Sunday night and wake up ready to go on Monday morning.

Of course, if you have problems with insomnia on Sunday nights, it also could be due to other things, such as Sunday afternoon football. Being a couch potato all afternoon can produce insomnia at night.

Naturally, we are not saying that everybody should go to bed early on Friday and Saturday nights or that nobody should sleep late on Saturday or Sunday mornings. There are many people who have no problem with Sunday night insomnia. Also, sometimes you may choose to stay up late to be with friends, knowing that you will have to pay for it with a difficult Monday morning. That's okay, as long as you understand that you're not struggling with serious insomnia, only a temporary confusion of your sleep-wake rhythm.

People Who Stay Up Late

A woman recently wrote to Ann Landers about having troubles being a night owl when everyone else she knew was a lark. She probably had *delayed sleep phase syndrome*. People with this syndrome simply have slow clocks, and they don't get sleepy until 3 or 4 in the morning because their body clock says it's only 10 or 11 P.M. They usually go to bed late—the woman who wrote to Ann Landers went to bed at 6 in the morning—and then stay in bed until noon or later.

We know of a retired government official who, now in his 70s, still has a very slow clock. All his life, he struggled with the need to get up around 7 A.M. when he felt he should sleep longer. Finally, retirement came. It was like heaven to be able to sleep every morning until 9 or 10 A.M. Unfortunately, after a few weeks of this great bliss, he developed extreme difficulties falling asleep. First, he could not fall asleep until 2 or 3 A.M., after which, naturally, he slept later in the morning. Then he couldn't fall asleep until 6 or 7 A.M. The later he fell asleep, of course, the longer he slept during the day. As he slept later and later, he did not get sleepy until later and later at night. By the time he came for help, he had an almost total day-night reversal.

Some people have clocks that are just a little slow. They are mild night owls who like the nighttime hours. But in some patients, the deviation is much more severe.

This was the case with Helen Roberts, a 26-year-old journalist who sought help for sleep-onset insomnia after she was fired because she overslept so regularly. She explained that she would lie in bed four to six hours before falling asleep and then would have extreme difficulty getting up the next day. Except for a certain defensiveness concerning her inability to arise on schedule, she seemed to be in good mental health.

Ms. Roberts had gone to extraordinary lengths to try to get up in the morning. She had asked friends to come in the morning and drag her to a cold shower. She had numerous alarm clocks that were so loud that they aroused the neighbors in her duplex (but not her). She tried to go to bed at a regular time, but no matter what she did, she simply could not fall asleep until the early morning hours. Even with the extraordinary measures she had taken, she could not make it to work on time. On Saturdays and Sundays, she slept "gloriously" from about 6 A.M. until late in the afternoon, and she felt excellent after these sleeps.

As part of a research study, Ms. Roberts was admitted to a time-free environment. Being a free-lance writer now, she took large amounts of work with her and wrote until she was tired, then relaxed for an hour or so and went to sleep. Miraculously, it seemed to her, her insomnia totally disappeared in the time-free environment, and she got incredible amounts of work done each day.

The surprise came when, at the end of the study, she was told how long she had been in the time-free environment. She thought it had been about 16 days; actually it had been 28 days. Typically, she had worked about 20 hours at a stretch and then slept for about 15 hours, making an average day/night of about 35 hours. She would have been just fine on a planet that rotated every 35 hours.

For a while, she tried to live a time-free lifestyle, simply going to bed and getting up whenever she felt like it. While this was a time of good sleep, high productivity, and a feeling of well-being, she became socially isolated. She would never know when she'd be sleeping on a certain day, and she couldn't plan any events in advance.

We'll tell you in a minute what solved her case.

Phototherapy: Treating a Fast or Slow Clock

In one startling study of 200 blind people, nine out of ten reported sleep disturbances. Most said that they were excessively sleepy during the day, had trouble falling asleep, or woke up frequently in the middle of the night. There also is a particularly high incidence of sleep disturbances in people who spend most of the time indoors or who live isolated lives.

Light is an important zeitgeber. For the person with a short or long sleep-wake rhythm, light treatment (phototherapy) can be very helpful.

Here's how it is administered: You sit three feet away from a bright light for one or two hours. It must be a very bright light, the intensity used being at least 2,500 lux (ordinary room light is 150 to 200 lux, and bright summer sunshine is 100,000 lux). Ordinary room light is not intense enough to produce any effect.

Typically, you start with about one hour of exposure to the very bright light. If the light makes you too "hyper," cut down the amount of light exposure to half an hour. If, on the other hand, there is no effect, then you might go to two hours. Do this every day.

One version of a phototherapy light is a light box mounted with eight fluorescent tubes. You can buy such lighting fixtures from Natural Lighting Products, Lake Hopatcong, NJ 07849; The Sun Box Company, 1037 Taft Street, Rockville, MD 20850; Ambulatory Monitoring, 731 Saw Mill River Road, Ardsley, NY 10502; Rocky Mountain Medical, 200 Apollo Road, Montrose, CO 81401; and Apollo Light Systems, 352 West 1060th South, Orem, UT 84058, among others.

You also can make a unit yourself. Buy four shop lights with two 4 foot fluorescent tubes each. Screw hooks into the rafters of the ceiling and hang the lights from the screws. Or you can make an easel-type frame with four lights on each side. A plastic diffuser in front of the lights helps to absorb the glare. Sit about two feet away from the light at the time of the day when your body wants to be asleep while you want to be awake. You can eat, read, or exercise, whatever you want. Just don't wear sunglasses, since the phototherapy works by acting on the retina of the eyes.

Within just a few days, there usually is improvement in sleep and you feel more alert at the desired time. But the phototherapy must be continued, because you may relapse in a few days if it is stopped. You might try keeping it up for a month, and then, if you are sure that your new sleep schedule is well entrenched, you might try stopping the phototherapy. See what happens without it to determine whether you need to continue it for a longer period.

Chronotherapy: Resetting Your Clock

If a person has a delayed clock—such as a teenager who has stayed up until 5 A.M. each night during the summer and now has to get back to school—there is a one-time treatment to reset the hands of the clock. The technique of changing your body's schedule is called *chronotherapy*. For most people the clock must be moved forward, not backward.

If you think chronotherapy might help you, try to make the change-over when you don't have to be at school or work at a regular time. The first night, don't go to bed at what has been your usual late bedtime—say, 5 A.M.—but move your schedule forward by three hours; go to bed, say, at 8 in the morning, and sleep as late as you feel like. The next day, go to bed three hours later—at 11 A.M.—and sleep until late afternoon or whenever. In about a week, you can "go around the clock" in this way so that you now go to bed at 10 or 11 in the evening.

Once you are at the time that you want to go to bed, you have to be very tough on yourself in getting up at the same time each morning. Otherwise, your clock will start going around the circle again. You also might want to start phototherapy in the morning to keep the clock fixed at the new time.

One student we know has always had problems getting up in the morning, but was able to stay reasonably on schedule for the nine months of college. In the summer, he worked on a night job because it was so much easier for him. His job started at 5 P.M. and ended at 1 in the morning, and after work he would hang out with his friends. By the end of the summer, he was going to bed between 6 and 7 in the morning and sleeping until 3 in the afternoon, then getting ready for work.

Now he was back in college and could not get used to the morning hours. He had already missed half the first semester's morning classes and was flunking.

He did chronotherapy over Thanksgiving vacation, doing it much faster than usual. On the first day, he slept from 5 in the morning until 2 in the afternoon. Then he moved forward five hours and slept from 10 in the morning until whenever he woke up. The next day, he went to sleep at 3 in the afternoon, and the next day at 7 in the evening; by the end of the holiday, his bedtime was 12 midnight—his desired bedtime.

This chronotherapy was very fast because he did not have much time, but he did it successfully. He was told to be very careful from then on never to sleep late, because his clock would run away from him again. As it turned out, if he stayed up late one night and slept late, the one night didn't seem to make a difference. But if he stayed up late two nights and slept late two mornings, then he had to go around the clock again.

The writer described earlier—Ms. Roberts—was treated with chronotherapy. She worked her way around the clock in four days. She then tried to hold her wake-up time constant at 7 A.M., which she could do for about two weeks. But during those two weeks, it would become harder and harder to fall asleep, until she slipped back into the old routine of staying up late and sleeping until the afternoon. Then she would do four days of chronotherapy again. In this way, she could predict when she would be on a normal 24-hour cycle, and she could block out the four or five days when she would be on her chronotherapy and keep social or business appointments properly scheduled.

Recently, Ms. Roberts also had bright lights installed in her study for phototherapy each morning. This has sped up her clock considerably, and she needs chronotherapy less often.

Cases as extreme as this are rare. Nevertheless, if your clock is not close to 24 hours, chronotherapy and phototherapy might be able to help reset your clock and control your rhythm.

Nobody is irretrievably stuck with their sleep-wake rhythm. Your rhythm can be changed. Some people prefer not to change their cycle, though, and just build their lives around it the way it is. One patient, a TV repairman, felt this way. He had a history of never going to bed until the middle of the night. He decided to arrange his job so that he could come into the TV shop in the evening and all night long repair the sets that had been dropped off during the day. He went home in the morning, and the day group came in and took care of the customers, who were happy with the fast overnight service.

So you can change your rhythm or you can live with it. But if you're an insomniac, you should do your best to keep it constant.

···· 12 ····

Night Work, Jet Lag, and Seasonal Affective Disorder (SAD)

There are three clock-related situations that can upset our sleep rhythms and cause problems. They are night work, jet lag, and seasonal affective disorder (SAD).

Working on the Night Shift

Humans are built to be night sleepers, not night workers. We have the biological potential to stay up and work during times when we should be sleeping, but in general our hormones and our rhythms are geared for daytime wakefulness.

However, modern civilization has grown into an all-day-and-all-night operation, unnaturally forcing many people to work at night. Some night work is unavoidable: We need security forces at night and hospitals to be open to care for the critically ill, and in some factories the equipment has to be on day and night for technical reasons. However, we have gone way beyond the necessary. It is not absolutely necessary for grocery stores to stay open all night, and all factories do not need to run 24 hours a day.

When we compute profits from round-the-clock operations, we often forget that there are serious human costs in shift work that do not reach the balance sheets.

Circadian rhythms are finely tuned phenomena in which hundreds of body functions mesh with each other. When we change work shifts, it takes time to reestablish that fine balance. It usually takes at least two weeks before we are fully adjusted to a total day-night reversal, unless we are artificially adjusted by exposure to very bright light.

It would not be that difficult to get used to permanent night-shift work, *if* we would be consistent about it. For Peter's own Ph.D. thesis, he stayed up nights and slept days for 45 consecutive days. After two weeks, he was totally habituated to the new schedule and felt as alert and well at night and slept as soundly during the day as he had before the day-night reversal. But this is not how shift work is usually done. Night-shift workers usually stay on the night shift for perhaps five days and then get two days off. During these two days, they want to be with their families, and they try to sleep at night and be awake during the day. Then another night shift begins, and they switch back. Because it takes about two weeks to adjust completely to a day-night reversal, permanent night-shift workers may never get totally habituated. They spend their lives, sometimes 40 years of it, in a permanent kind of jet lag.

Under these circumstances, mood deteriorates. Performance goes down dramatically, and there are health consequences. For example, digestive secretions follow a circadian pattern. If you eat while on the night shift, you fill your stomach with food at the time when it is not ready for digestion, and you leave it empty when all the acid secretions occur. This probably is why shift workers have more peptic ulcers than nonshift workers do.

Shift work does not affect all people equally. It is easiest on night owls and on people who are good sleepers, though it increases stress and disrupts family life even in them. Shiftwork is hardest on insomniacs. Even if society does not address the problem, you can keep your own sleep problem in mind when you make any decision about whether or not to do shift work.

Working five nights a week and then changing the schedule to be with one's family on weekends is bad enough, but what may be even worse is working rotating shifts of one week on night shift, one week on evening shift, and one week on day shift. Workers on rotating one-week shifts always are out of step with their rhythms. It is much better to have longer shift-rotation periods, say three weeks. During the night shift, you probably show disrupted rhythms because you work five days, then take two days off to be with your family. But during the three weeks each of morning and evening shift, you can sleep a normal schedule of about midnight to about 6 A.M. This gives you six weeks to get synchronized. Therefore, three-week rotations are much less detrimental to health than are one-week rotations.

Another factor can help to reduce the sleep-cycle disruption caused by shift work. Often, the rotation of shifts is a week on the morning shift (7 A.M. to 3 P.M.), followed by a week on the night shift (11 P.M. to 7 A.M.), followed by a week on the evening shift (3 to 11 P.M.). Because shift workers usually are younger, they often have slow clocks; therefore, the rotation should go: morning shift, evening shift, night shift. Shifts should be moved forward around the clock, not backward. (However, for the person over about age 55, who usually has a fast clock, the shifts would be better reversed—a week of night shift, then evening shift, then morning shift.)

Dr. Charles Czeisler and his colleagues at the Center for the Design of Industrial Schedules at Harvard Medical School did a study of shift work among members of the Philadelphia police force. They looked into the benefits of trying to modify police work schedules to fit these principles of circadian rhythms.

When the study began, the officers worked six consecutive days followed by two days off, then changed shifts counterclockwise: from morning to night to evening—just the opposite of what is recommended. Czeisler's team found that more than half the police officers reported at least a moderate problem with poor sleep, a quarter said they had been involved in an automobile accident or near-miss from sleepiness in the past year, and 80 percent said that they had fallen asleep at least once a week during night-shift duty.

An alternative schedule assigned shifts to rotate clockwise and lengthened the time between shift changes from 8 to 18 days. Reports of poor sleep dropped by more than a third, and daytime tiredness went from 40 percent to 20 percent. On-the-job motor-vehicle accidents dropped from 50 to 30 per million miles driven. Use of sleeping pills and alcohol was cut in half.

Industry studies show that similar changes in scheduling can increase manufacturing productivity. In a three-month trial with one company, Dr. Richard Coleman, of Stanford University Medical School, showed that productivity improved by 20 percent when shifts were rotated forward with the clock and lasted no less than three weeks. The study also showed a "dramatic improvement in job satisfaction, schedule satisfaction, and health improvement in the workers." So it is to the advantage of both the company and the workers to change to saner shift schedules.

At the 1989 annual meeting of the Association of Professional Sleep Societies in Washington, DC, Dr. Czeisler and Dr. Richard Kronauer, of Harvard, reported success in readjusting the biological clocks of 14 men, aged 18 to 24. They exposed the men to five hours of bright light for three consecutive days at the time their body temperature was lowest (the time that people are sleepiest). The third exposure to light restarted their day-night cycle as if it were daytime, regardless of the actual time. This could mean that by using bright light, you could make the readjustment to a new shift time in three days instead of the usual two weeks.

Dangers to the Public

There has been so much concern about the dangers to the public caused by workers being sleepy on the job that several groups have made major studies of the problem. Assistant Secretary for Health and Human Services Dr. James Mason says the issue is of increasing public and legislative concern.

One important analysis was reported in 1987 by the Association of Professional Sleep Societies. Its Committee on Catastrophes, Sleep and Public Policy found that almost everyone has an increased tendency to sleep and a diminished capacity to function during the early morning hours from about 2 to 7 A.M. and, to a lesser degree, during midafternoon from about 2 to 5 P.M. Fatigue is most likely to hit us at these times and, if we have been deprived of sleep, the letdown will be greater at these times. The association's committee urges policy makers in the fields of labor, management, and government to be alert to the problem.

Committee chairman Dr. Merrill Mitler, scientific director of the Scripps Clinic Sleep Disorders Center in La Jolla, California, says that the accumulated data suggest that employers may be "asking too much of the human body . . . they think that if the pay is high enough and management strong enough, they will have alert workers. We've shown that that's dangerous thinking."

Sleepiness can be very hazardous to your health, as well as to the health of others. Dr. John K. Lauber, of the National Transportation Safety Board, presented a special report on the problem at the 1988

Professional Sleep Societies meeting. His conclusion: "We have investigated many accidents in which sleep loss, sleep disorders, fatigue, and circadian factors are clearly implicated. I don't think we have the foggiest notion of the true prevalence of these factors in transportation system accidents. . . . Frequently, we find horror stories." For example: At 4 A.M. on April 13, 1984, two freight trains collided head-on at Wiggins, Colorado. Seven locomotives and 40 cars were derailed, and five crew members were killed. The National Transportation Safety Board determined that the probable cause of the accident was that the engineer and other crew members on one of the trains were asleep and failed to comply with restrictive signals.

On May 31, 1985, a northbound semitrailer collided with a southbound car and a school bus in North Carolina. Of the 27 school-bus passengers, 6 died and 12 sustained serious injuries. The truckdriver had had 1-1/2 hours of sleep during the 36 hours before the accident.

The three nuclear disasters—Three Mile Island, Peachtree, and Chernobyl—all happened in the early morning. Human error was cited as a factor in all three. Was sleepiness also a factor? Did people make the mistakes because they were either sleeping or very sleepy?

The Airline Pilots Association adds that an upset in biorhythms and inadequate rest can affect a pilot's judgment and may have contributed to several major accidents. To avoid further tragedies, rules for pilot flight time, rest time, and shift schedules must take circadian rhythms into account, they say.

It pays to be asleep between 2 and 7 A.M. It's best for the worker and it's best for the public. At those times, especially during quiet pursuits such as driving or sitting at a control panel, sleepiness may prove overwhelming. And the greater the sleep debt, the more likely a person is to inadvertently slip into sleep. It's a myth that people know their limits; if you think you're going to know when it's time to pull over and sleep, you may be fatally wrong.

How To Sleep Better If You're Doing Shift Work

Obviously, if you are a poor sleeper, it would be best if you didn't have to do shift work at all. However, if it is unavoidable, here are some things you can do.

When you come home after work, give yourself plenty of time to slow down before going to bed. You cannot expect to work until 11 P.M. and then fall asleep by 11:30.

Schedule your sleep time and defend it vigorously. If you work night shift and sleep from 8 A.M. to 2 P.M., do not get up if a neighbor happens to drop in at 11 A.M. for a friendly chat. Dropping in at that time on a shift worker is as rude as dropping in on a day worker at 4 A.M.

Make your bedroom as dark and as soundproof as possible. Try to sleep where there is not a lot of family activity or a noisy kitchen or bathroom nearby. Earplugs and sleeping masks may help.

Limit the amount of coffee, tea, and cola you drink. Drink it only at the beginning of your shift. When you eat at night, avoid heavy, spicy, or hard-to-digest foods.

If you work on a rotating shift, try preparing for your new sleep schedule on your days off before the shift changes. When your next shift is the evening shift, try staying up a little later at night and sleeping later in the morning to ease into the new schedule.

Plan some quality time with your family and friends for exercise, relaxation, and fun, and set up a definite schedule committed to those times. If you're married, talk to your spouse about your special needs. Many shift workers have told us that support and understanding at home are the most important aspects of adjusting successfully to shift work. You need to talk about how you can adjust your life to your unusual work times. For shift workers, as well as for other people, it is a good idea to set aside some regular time each week to talk about what is going on in your lives as a result of your work hours and to learn what is going on in your family's lives when you are not there. Plan some special events for your days off. Taking a son or daughter alone with you to a sports event or on a shopping trip could mean much more to you and your child than a few nights together in front of the television set.

Jet Lag and How to Avoid It

Jet lag occurs when you travel quickly across several time zones, causing your internal biological rhythm to be out of sync with the new local time. At the destination, you feel tired and washed out. Despite the fatigue, sleep is riddled with many awakenings and is not restorative. Some three out of four travelers have jet lag, according to one study. Your brain is foggy, you have trouble concentrating, you become irritable, your reactions are slow, and you may have stomach and intestinal problems.

A minor form of jet lag occurs in some people even during the change to or from daylight saving time. While some people take the one-hour switch in stride, others take up to a week to feel comfortable.

Jet lag becomes especially noticeable after crossing three or more time zones; for example, flying from Hawaii to New York. Most people, especially young people with their slower-than-24-hour circadian rhythms, have an easier time flying from east to west and a harder time going from west to east, because that means squeezing their long body-clock time into a day that is shorter than 24 hours. Older people sometimes have the opposite problem: more difficulty going from east to west.

(There is no jet lag when flying north and south, because the time zone is the same from the North Pole to the South Pole.)

Studies have been done on overseas-traveling businesspersons, pilots, stewardesses, actors, chess players, athletes, and even race-horses. After crossing many time zones on an eastward or westward flight, none of them functioned at optimal levels for the first few days, not even the racehorses. Just when you arrive for an important appointment, when you would like to be sharp and alert, your body is rebelling and adjusting. The problem can be crucial for a diplomat or business executive who, on arrival, will be making important decisions. (Henry Kissinger writes in *White House Years* that he had some problems at the Vietnam peace negotiations because he attended them immediately after a long plane flight.)

If a meeting is important, get to your destination several days early to allow your body to adjust. If it is necessary to hold meetings during the first day or two of a visit, try to schedule them at times when you would be awake and alert at home. An American in England might schedule meetings in late afternoon for the first days, for example, since that would correspond to morning work hours in the United States. A morning appointment would feel like the middle of the night.

You can help to prevent jet lag if, before you leave home, you gradually adjust your hours of sleeping and eating to the time zone of your destination. For example, if you are going to fly from New York to California, you might go to bed later and later over several days until you go to bed and get up close to California time. Eat your meals close to the time that you'll be eating them in California. Even if it is not convenient to change completely to the new time before you go, at least you can reschedule your day somewhat in that direction.

On the plane, drink plenty of fluids to help prevent dehydration from the low humidity in the airplane. Dehydration seems to make it more difficult for the body's rhythms to adjust. Also, if you are worried about jet lag, don't smoke or drink alcohol or much caffeine, which add further stress to your system.

When you get to your destination, switch immediately to the new time. Do not go to bed just because you're tired, but wait until it is appropriate for the new time zone. Go outside, even if you are tired, and walk, sit in a park, or eat at a sidewalk cafe and soak up as much sunshine as possible. On the second day, go out in the sun again as much as possible. On the third day, with the coming of daylight, your body clock should be reset to local time.

Drs. Roger Cole and Daniel Kripke of San Diego reported at the 1989 meeting of the Association of Professional Sleep Societies that their research indicates that getting sunlight early in the morning is best if you want to wake up earlier in the day (you flew from west to east), and getting sunlight in the late afternoon and evening is best if you want to wake up later in the morning (you flew from east to west). (If you forgot which way is correct, when your body wants to sleep and you want to stay awake, go out in the sun.)

Dr. Mitsuo Sasaki, of Tokyo, reported at the same meeting that Japan Air Lines has set up a special, brightly lit room in San Francisco for a group of pilots so they could use phototherapy to help them reset their body clocks and avoid jet lag. Subjects also took vitamin B12 for two weeks before their flight and for one week afterward, which Dr. Sasaki said enhanced their response to the light and made it work better.

About two decades ago, the U.S. Army needed to demonstrate to its NATO allies that it was capable of transporting whole troop divisions from America to Europe and having them combat-ready within 24 hours. This was done, and the U.S. servicemen engaged in maneuvers immediately after they had landed in Germany. To everyone's surprise, the U.S. infantrymen adjusted to the European time zone within about two days, while their commanding officers still suffered terribly from jet lag two weeks later. Outdoor light and activity are powerful zeitgebers, as discussed in the previous chapter, and readjust our internal clocks with great efficiency. The infantrymen had plenty of both. The officers, sitting in dimly lit bunkers, did not have zeitgebers. This is why we stressed earlier when you travel, get plenty of light and activity as soon as you can.

Recently, a number of diets have been proposed to help with jet lag. Most recommend that you feast one day and hunger the next, to make the body ready for the time-zone jump. We have not been too impressed that these diets really work. (However, in the spirit of our program, you may wish to try them for yourself.) It is more likely that, in a few years, airplane passengers will walk around with big goggles that give them bright light at the time they will need to be awake at their new destination and dim light at the new time they will have to be sleeping.

Other research has been geared to the use of the chemical melatonin, a hormone that is inhibited by light. Preliminary results indicate that giving melatonin to people at specific times each day for several days before a long flight may reduce jet-lag symptoms. Melatonin also has promise as a sleeping pill of the future to help patients who need adjustments of their circadian clocks.

Do You Sleep Longer and Get Depressed in the Winter?

In the early 1980s, Dr. Peter S. Mueller, a psychiatrist at the National Institute of Mental Health, was treating a 29-year-old woman for cyclic bouts of winter depression. Over several years, the patient moved to a number of different cities. Mueller maintained contact with her and observed that the farther north she lived, the earlier in the fall she became depressed and the longer she stayed depressed in the spring. When she traveled to the Caribbean in midwinter, her depression disappeared within days. Mueller began to speculate that the lack of sunlight was involved in some way with the woman's depression and decided to test that theory. On consecutive mornings, he exposed her to bright, full-spectrum light. In less than a week, she recovered from her depression.

Mueller's findings came to the attention of Drs. Norman Rosenthal, Thomas Wehr, and Alfred Lewy, who also were interested in depression. They launched a full-scale investigation into winter depression, recruiting large numbers of volunteers for observation and treatment.

This was the beginning of the understanding of what is now called seasonal affective disorder, or SAD.

The classic symptoms include depression, lethargy, and prolonged sleep, combined with bouts of carbohydrate craving and overeating. Sufferers go to sleep early and stay in bed for nine or ten hours, and their sleep is intermittent and not fully refreshing. During the day, SAD patients often are drowsy and have trouble concentrating. There also is a craving for light. Such people go around their homes turning on as many lights as they can (usually only to have the rest of the family turn them all off again to save electricity).

The symptoms appear in the late fall or early winter and last until the following spring. Once spring arrives, SAD patients are full of energy, creativity, and zest for life, and their cravings for carbohydrates lessen.

There seem to be a number of factors involved in SAD: the hormone melatonin, which affects mood and energy levels (and is suppressed by light); the chemical serotonin, which is involved with the nervous system and also regulates a person's appetite for carbohydrate-rich foods; and the first of the two "oscillators"—or time clocks—in the body, the one that is governed by light.

In some people, the winter months in cold climates do not provide enough light to regulate that oscillator. It then becomes "free-running," which could explain the upsets in sleep that occur in patients with SAD.

The answer, for many patients, is to take as long a vacation as possible to a sunny place in the winter.

Others find relief using phototherapy (discussed in detail in the previous chapter). Light exposure in the morning, according to some investigators, seems to be more effective than light exposure later in the day; other researchers say whether the light is given in the morning or afternoon doesn't make any difference. Patients need to check it out for themselves. Also, the more intense the light, the shorter the exposure one seems to need. Many patients need one to two hours of exposure at 2,500 lux, but some need only 30 minutes at 10,000 lux.

If you don't want to spend the money for a light box, try sitting or walking in the sunshine for an hour each day. Dr. Anna Wirz-Justice of Basel, Switzerland, reported at the 1989 meeting of the Association of Professional Sleep Societies that, done regularly, this worked just as well in a group of her patients.

A typical patient was Kate Norris, a 38-year-old farmer's wife with two children. She worked on the farm all summer long, from sunup to sundown. But when the harvest was in, from about Thanksgiving on, she typically went into hibernation. Both she and her husband thought she simply was overworked from the summer and needed a few months to rest. Usually, by planting time, she was up and active again.

Then the farm crisis hit and, after a valiant struggle, the couple lost their farm and moved into town. Mrs. Norris worked as a waitress, which she did not find especially exhausting, but, to her surprise, she went into the same "hibernation" that year as she had on the farm. She barely could get herself up to go to work, and her children and husband were left to manage their home during the winter.

This lasted for three years, with one major exception. As a prize for good performance on the job, her husband won a cruise for two to the Bahamas. To her great surprise, Mrs. Norris recovered her zest for living after the first two days on the cruise ship. But sleepiness came back a few days after she returned home.

Since the second year in town, Mrs. Norris had consulted a psychiatrist off and on when she felt depressed and tired. Various antidepressants were tried, but none helped. However, when her psychiatrist heard of her recovery on the cruise ship, he diagnosed SAD and prescribed bright lights. Her husband rigged a light station where she could sit every morning for an hour. She read or ate breakfast at her light station, and within two weeks, her depression and excessive sleep were gone. Indeed, she became somewhat hyperactive, so the light exposure was decreased to 40 minutes.

Over the next two years, Mrs. Norris spent about 40 minutes each morning at her light station from about November to March. Excessive sleeping and depression are things of the past.

Several studies show that, no matter where they live, many people get less than an hour of sunlight during their average day. It might well improve our sleep, as well as our moods, if most of us, especially people with indoor jobs and lifestyles, arranged to be outside more and exposed to more light.

···· 13 ····

Medical Causes

Brenda's husband, Scott, had no trouble sleeping in their apartment, but when they went to Brenda's parents' summer cottage for a short vacation every fall, Scott would toss and turn most of the night and sleep half the day away. Brenda accused him of not wanting to spend time with her parents. The truth was that Scott had an allergy to cat dander, and Brenda's parents had a cat. When he tried to escape by going outside, there was ragweed in the air, and he was allergic to that, too. He slept poorly at night and was tired all day because of the allergies.

Scott's brother, Bob, had a problem, too. After an operation on his knee, he developed arthritis. Whenever his knee did not get enough exercise, Bob was awake at night with pain.

These are two examples of how medical conditions can cause insomnia. If you have not been able to overcome your insomnia with all the guidelines we have given you so far, you should consider seeing your physician for a medical checkup.

Sometimes, the medical cause of poor sleep is obvious. For example, pain from arthritis, a toothache, a headache, or a sore muscle might keep anyone awake. Other times, a medical cause may not be so obvious. For example, some infections can cause insomnia. And maybe it's not a medical condition itself that causes a sleep problem, but a medication that's being taken.

· · · · ● · · ·

Anthony, a 26-year-old graduate student in zoology, woke up frequently each night and was tired much of the day. He was worried, because his Ph.D. exam was coming up in a few months, and in his present state he simply was too exhausted to prepare for it. He had always been a high achiever, graduating fourth in his college class, and the thought of failing his Ph.D. exam frightened him. He had frequent nightmares in which he would see himself flunking.

He was so clearly a nervous wreck that for once I abandoned my usual requirement that patients have a thorough physical exam before coming for behavioral treatment. I taught him relaxation training, better management skills, and better sleep hygiene. He became calmer and more focused, but his nightly awakenings persisted. So I went back to the basics and did what I should have done at the beginning: I took a thorough history—and found the key.

About six months earlier, Anthony had taken a summer course studying tropical wildlife in Brazil. There he had had a "feverish cold" that had sapped his strength for the last two weeks in Brazil.

I not only sent Anthony for a general medical exam, but also referred him to a specialist in tropical diseases. A tropical parasite was discovered and treated. His sleep improved, and while Anthony claimed that my teachings in stress management helped him pass his exams, I was embarrassed and resolved never again to rush into behavioral treatment without first assessing the entire person, no matter how obvious the case seemed.

· · · ● ● ● · ·

Medical Conditions That Can Cause Sleep Problems

There are many medical conditions that can cause insomnia. Asthma can cause coughing, and allergies can cause a stuffed nose or itching eyes. Bronchitis and emphysema can cause breathing difficulties, heart trouble can cause chest pain or difficulty in breathing, digestive problems can cause heartburn, and abnormalities in swallowing can cause coughing and gagging. An ulcer or arthritis can cause pain. A urinary-tract infection can trigger frequent waking. Itching from insect bites or hives can keep a person awake. The hot flashes of menopause can wake a woman up. Indeed, almost any medical disorder can cause either insomnia or excessive daytime sleepiness in some patients.

Other, hidden medical causes include such things as an infection, a brain tumor, parkinsonism, kidney disease, thyroid problems, or a metabolic disorder such as diabetes. Poor sleep can be caused by alcoholism or drug abuse. Even low estrogen levels after menopause can cause insomnia (often improved with estrogen-replacement therapy). Other possible causes of insomnia include anemia; carbon-monoxide poisoning; multiple sclerosis; poisoning with arsenic, mercury, copper, or other heavy metals; or side effects of radiation or chemotherapy.

And don't forget mental illness. As we pointed out in Chapter 2, insomnia is one of the symptoms of depression or other mental illnesses. Depressed patients often wake up early in the morning, but usually have no trouble falling asleep at night. You should talk to your doctor if you think depression might be a possible cause of your insomnia, especially if you also have lost you appetite, have lost interest in daily life, and feel lonely or hopeless.

In children, the most common medical causes of poor sleep are teething, gastrointestinal disorders, tonsil and adenoid enlargement, pain from colic, pain from joint disease and worms. (If your child has trouble getting to sleep, is restless, and scratches the anus, be suspicious of worms and consult the child's doctor.) More rarely, chorea, encephalitis, and rickets can cause insomnia in children. Other common causes are pain and irritation from wet bedclothes and poor behavioral training by parents.

There's one good thing about finding that a medical problem is the cause of your insomnia: When the medical condition is treated, the poor sleep usually is cured. Once depression, for example, is treated, problems with insomnia usually improve greatly. In fact, when a depressed patient has an improvement in sleep, it is often used as a sign that recovery from the depression has begun.

Could any of these conditions be causing your sleep problem? If you think it's possible, discuss it with your doctor so that you can receive proper treatment and get back to sleep sound again.

Sleep Disorders of Pregnancy

Most women in the first trimester (three months) of pregnancy are very sleepy during the daytime. This often is the first sign of pregnancy, even before morning sickness occurs. Daytime sleepiness early in pregnancy may be caused by an increase in the hormone progesterone, which is known to have a sedative effect.

Later in pregnancy, women may have difficulty sleeping because they simply can't get comfortable. But no matter how uncomfortable you might be, *do not take any sleeping medications*, even over-the-counter ones. Don't even use alcohol to get to sleep. *Any* drug or medication can possibly harm your baby. Instead, use behavioral techniques such as those outlined in the chapters on relaxation (Chapter 7) and stress (Chapter 8).

Sundowner's Syndrome and Medical Problems of Aging

As the brain ages, some people seem to need more stimulation to keep functioning normally and rationally. Some older people, especially those with mild forms of senile dementia, remain oriented and function acceptably during the day, but with nightfall, stimulation decreases, and they become agitated and confused. This is called *sundowner's syndrome.*

Another problem in older people is that medications are metabolized more slowly. Often, what used to be an adequate dose is now an overdose. For example, sleeping pills that used to be metabolized adequately during the eight hours of sleep now may remain in the system twice as long, causing daytime sedation. Pills that might have a side effect of mild insomnia in a 30-year-old could cause severe insomnia in a 70-year-old.

Beginning in their late 40s or their 50s, most people don't sleep as soundly as they used to. They wake more often during the night and stay awake longer, and doze off more easily during the day. Some older people have dozens of little awakenings at night, lasting perhaps 15 seconds or less. This sometimes gives people the impression that they have been awake all night, even though they haven't been. (Recognizing this possibility usually helps make the feeling more bearable.)

If you are past middle age and are sleeping poorly, consider that some of these factors could be having an effect on you.

There are two rules to practice when you get old enough to retire. One: Don't sit around doing nothing all day. You must have enough stimulation and activity during the day to have good sleep at night. Two: Don't make a habit of turning over and going back to sleep in the morning. It may seem like one of the privileges of retirement—

but if you are an insomniac, it is a mistake. It makes it more difficult to fall asleep the next night, and soon you have started a vicious circle.

This was the case with Duke Franconi, who had worked as a shipping clerk during the day and a part-time bartender at night. He slept well until he retired, giving up both jobs at about the same time. He felt like a king for a few weeks, not having to get up in the morning to go to the loading dock and being able to go to bed whenever he wanted. However, about three months after retirement, he developed serious insomnia. He was wide awake every night from midnight until morning and soon started taking sleeping pills. After awhile, they didn't work anymore, and he came to the sleep lab for advice.

Taking his history, it became clear that Mr. Franconi, before his retirement, had slept only about six hours per night, from about 11 P.M. til 5 A.M., and he had felt that this was satisfactory. He had not needed to sleep later on weekends.

Now, Mr. Franconi was taking a one-hour nap in the morning "because I didn't sleep last night." He also took an afternoon nap from 4 to 6 P.M. and usually was so sleepy after dinner that he retired around 8 P.M. But at midnight he was wide awake and unable to sleep!

Adding the hours, it was clear that Mr. Franconi now slept a total of seven hours, one hour more than he had before retirement. He didn't need sleeping pills—he needed less sleep. He was sleeping an hour too much.

We tried to convince Mr. Franconi to give up his morning and afternoon naps and go to bed later. This would have consolidated his sleep and permitted him to sleep after midnight. However, he felt that he had worked all his life and deserved to rest whenever he felt like it. And he still wanted sleeping pills.

Then help came from an unexpected source. His divorced daughter, raising two preschoolers, had a car accident and was laid up in the hospital for more than a month. Tough Duke had to take care of the children. They kept him hopping all day! Once they were in bed, he had barely time to unwind before, totally exhausted, he fell into a sound sleep. At first it was hard, but after three weeks of a forced regular sleep-wake cycle, he felt so good he swore he'd never go back to his old lazy retirement days again.

Obviously, many factors were involved here. Duke felt needed again, instead of useless. And being around young children can be invigorating. But the most crucial factor was that he got back to a regular sleep-wake rhythm.

Poisoning from Toxic Metals

Insomnia or excessive sleepiness in the daytime also may be symptoms of acute poisoning with heavy metals or other poisons.

An article in the *Archives of Environmental Health* describes the effects of exposure to lead among lead-acid-battery factory workers. Half of 92 exposed workers had insomnia, fatigue, weakness, and drowsiness. Another study in the same journal showed similar sleep disturbances, fatigue, and weakness in 680 copper-smelter workers from lead and arsenic exposure. Sleep disorders and fatigue also were found in a study of 1,200 people living in a small city in West Germany where they were exposed to the metal thallium emitted by a nearby cement plant. The thallium, found by urine and hair tests, had been picked up from vegetables and fruit grown in gardens that were exposed to cement dust fallout.

Sometimes, exposure to toxic metals is not obvious. For example, Mary Louise Megan was an avid tennis player and energetic housewife in the midwest when her husband was transferred to Los Angeles several years ago. After a few months, she developed headaches, insomnia, and fatigue and also found that she no longer had the coordination to play a decent game of tennis. A complete physical examination showed a high level of lead in her body. Further investigation revealed that she and her husband had bought a house along the freeway so that he could commute to work more easily. Her constant exposure to car and truck exhaust fumes had caused her to have a hidden, low-level lead poisoning. After she took medications plus a proper balance of beneficial mineral supplements, the lead was excreted more efficiently from her body and she felt good again.

Constant sleepiness and lethargy also can be the first signs of lead poisoning in children who may have gotten lead in their systems by eating flecks of paint or sucking icicles contaminated with lead. People working in industrial settings that routinely use toxic chemicals and heavy metals also are much at risk.

If you suspect that you could have been exposed to lead or other metals at work or at home, you can be tested for them by analysis of urine and by hair mineral.

Medicines May Be Hazardous to Your Sleep

A few years ago, a group of sleep researchers were talking about their patients who had insomnia as a side effect from various medications, and what could be done to help them. Said one: "I swear, the first thing we should do for most patients is to grab them by the feet and shake them until all the pills fall out of their pockets." That's how often medications can be the cause of poor sleep.

If you really need a certain medication, you might have to take it, no matter what. Often, however, there are alternative treatments for the same disease, with fewer or different side effects. For example, for depression, there are drugs such as Elavil that make you sleepy. If you take one of these drugs at night, you'll probably sleep well. Other antidepressants, such as Vivactil, tend to make you more alert. Still others have no influence on sleep.

Above all, beware of "escalating polypharmacy." It can happen quickly—you take one drug for a medical problem, a second one to combat the first one's side effects, a third one that another doctor gives you for the side effects of the second, and so on. Sometimes polypharmacy is necessary, but we see it more often than we should. If you're seeing more than one physician, each one may be prescribing medications without knowing about medicines you're getting from another.

Many prescription drugs and over-the-counter medications can cause sleep problems. For example, insomnia can be caused by medications for such things as asthma, thyroid disorders, and weight-reduction.

Here are some common insomnia-causing drugs:

- Several antidepressant drugs, especially mononamine-oxidase inhibitors
- Any drug with amphetamine, such as prescription diet pills
- Some drugs for high blood pressure
- Some birth control pills, although this is rare
- Bronchodilating drugs, such as for asthma, that contain ephedrine, aminophylline, or norepinephrine
- Caffeine-containing medications
- Sleeping pills and tranquilizers (insomnia may result from withdrawal on the nights when you are not using them)
- Steroid preparations
- Some thyroid preparations
- Some cancer chemotherapeutic agents

- Adrenocorticotropic hormone (ACTH)
- dopa for parkinsonism

These drugs can affect sleep in three major ways: They can cause difficulty in falling asleep, can cause sleep to be interrupted frequently, or can cause early morning awakenings.

If you suspect that a medication could be causing your insomnia, read the label. Does it contain amphetamine or caffeine? If so, the chances are strong that this medication is causing your sleep disturbances. Be particularly alert about painkillers. Since pain, no matter what the source, can keep us awake at night, it is tempting to take a painkiller to alleviate the pain so we can go to sleep. However, some of the painkillers contain caffeine, which can do more to keep you awake than the pain can.

In addition to reading the label, if a package insert came with the medication, read it also and see if it lists any sleep disturbances as possible side effects. If there is no package insert, call your pharmacist and ask him or her to check a reference for possible sleep side effects.

You also need to think about drug interactions. Perhaps a single drug alone would not cause you to have insomnia, but two drugs acting together might. If you are taking more than one drug regularly, check with your physician or pharmacist about possible drug interactions.

Warning: If it appears likely that a medication could be causing your trouble, do not stop taking it on your own. Call your physician to discuss the problem. The answer may be to change the dosage or to try another similar medication that does not disturb sleep. These are decisions that must be made by a physician knowledgable about the drug and about your particular case.

The Effects of Marijuana and Other Illegal Drugs

The most active compound in marijuana is delta-9 tetrahydrocannabinol (THC). This compound alters brain chemicals involved in sleep and produces changes in brain-wave patterns. According to the Association of Sleep Disorders Centers, long term marijuana use increases the time needed to get to sleep and reduces REM sleep. It is *not* a good sleep aid.

Cocaine is a stimulant that produces a sense of euphoria followed, in several hours, by a sense of depression. Its arousing and addictive properties stem from its effects on a chemical in the brain called dopamine, which is involved in sleep and wakefulness. Sleep changes caused by cocaine include insomnia, with both reduced deep sleep stages and reduced REM sleep. When cocaine is discontinued, the person becomes very sleepy and may feel that more cocaine is necessary just to function. Cocaine is particularly addictive when used in the very short-acting form known as crack.

Amphetamine and amphetamine-like drugs (also known as speed or crank) are powerful stimulants that are similar to cocaine in many respects. They, too, potentiate brain chemicals involved in wakefulness and produce changes in brain-wave patterns. Amphetamine-type drugs cause reduced delta (deep) sleep and reduced REM sleep, as well as a decreased tendency to fall asleep and stay asleep. As with cocaine, when amphetamine is discontinued, the person becomes very sleepy and may feel that more amphetamine is necessary just to function. Also, discontinuation of amphetamine leads to greatly increased REM sleep, known as *REM rebound* which may be accompanied by nightmares. (However, amphetamine and related drugs sometimes are medically useful in controlling the disabling daytime sleepiness of some sleep disorders such as narcolepsy.)

Heroin is a depressant. It retards both intellectual functioning and motor functioning, and it slows breathing. It decreases deep sleep and REM sleep. It also disturbs sleep by causing frequent shifts to stage 1 sleep and wakefulness. When discontinued, there can be withdrawal symptoms such as intense pain and extreme craving for more heroin. During withdrawal from heroin, there also may be REM rebound, accompanied by terrible nightmares.

You Need More Sleep to Fight Off Sickness

For centuries, our physicians and mothers have advised us to get plenty of rest to recover from an illness, and that's just what most patients feel like doing. Research now shows that our bodies really do crave more sleep when we are sick and that getting more sleep really does help.

Most people experience increased sleepiness when they have an infection. Interestingly, a substance similar to that found in certain bacteria has now been shown to promote sleep. Called *factor S,* this substance also stimulates production of interleukin-1 and interferon— key substances in immunity.

The newest evidence concerning the relationship between sleep and immune functions comes from the laboratory of Dr. Harvey Moldofsky, professor of psychiatry and medicine at Toronto Western Hospital. He found that in both animals and humans, interleukin is more active during delta (deep) sleep than at any other time of day or night. Perhaps vulnerability to disease is decreased and healing is speeded during delta sleep. It was found that when one injects tuberculin into normal subjects around 11 P.M., just before they get a large amount of delta sleep, there is less of an inflammatory reaction than if it is injected at 7 A.M. When ten men were kept awake in the sleep lab for 40 hours, their immune responses were considerably weaker after the sleep deprivation than after normal nights.

Physical Conditions That Your Doctor Wouldn't Know About

There are a number of things that cannot be diagnosed in a doctor's office because they occur only at night when you are asleep. In fact, chances are you don't know about them yourself, because you're asleep when they happen.

Here is what you can do: Ask your bed partner or another person to stay up a few hours and observe you while you are sleeping. You may be astonished at the findings.

For example, your observer may discover that you are one of the many people who wake up a lot because they are having problems with apnea. These stopped-breathing episodes may last 10 to 90 seconds. They often occur only when you sleep in certain positions (for example, on your back), or only in certain sleep phases (for example, in REM sleep), or only while you are falling asleep. Most of us have an occasional stopped-breathing episode, which you need not worry about. You do need to be concerned if you have to gasp for air repeatedly (more than fifteen times an hour, on average). This is called *sleep apnea syndrome*. If your friend observes many stopped-breathing episodes, discuss them with your doctor or seek help from a sleep disorders center.

The other problem that your partner may discover is periodic limb movement (PLM) during sleep. It can be your arms, but usually it is your legs that twitch or move about every 10 to 40 seconds. Sometimes, these movements can go on all night, or they may occur in episodes lasting only a few minutes.

We'll talk about apnea, nighttime twitching, restless legs, and other special sleep disorders in Chapter 15.

An Important Thing to Remember

Even if you find that your insomnia is caused by a medical condition or a medicine that you are taking for a medical condition, and you get that problem corrected, there still could be a further problem with sleeplessness.

If the insomnia caused by the medical condition has continued long enough, you may have learned bad habits—you may have become too worried about sleep and begun to associate sleeping with tension and frustration, as we discussed in Chapter 6. Even if a magic wand were to take away the disease that was causing the insomnia, you still might have insomnia, because now you have learned these bad habits.

So you need to treat everything medical that can possibly be treated, but you also may need to do some relearning by going back to Chapter 6 and reviewing the material on how you can build the right new habits for sleeping fit.

···· 14 ····

How to Kick the Sleeping Pill Habit

At one time, sleeping pills and tranquilizers were the most widely prescribed medications in the world. Now, thankfully, most physicians no longer are giving them out like sugar pills, but are prescribing them more selectively and for shorter times.

But sleeping pills are still overprescribed, in our judgment. Not one sleeping-pill manufacturer claims that sleeping pills should be used every night on a long term basis, yet many physicians still write prescriptions that way. And, of course, millions of over-the-counter sleeping pills are sold to anyone without prescription in pharmacies and grocery stores.

According to a special report issued in 1979 by the Institute of Medicine—National Academy of Sciences, sleeping pills may be more dangerous and less useful than either physicians or patients realize. To everyone's credit, sleeping-pill prescriptions have dropped from about 42 million in 1971 to the latest figure of about 21 million per year, but the report's warnings are still valid. Refills are still granted too casually, and millions of people still take the pills nightly for long periods.

Let's examine some of the facts that are now known about sleeping pills.

Sleeping Pills Work Only for a Short Time

Sleeping pills are not effective for as long as most people think they are. The older sleeping pills, such as barbiturates, often lose their effectiveness after one or two weeks. The newer pills may remain effective for a few months, but certainly not for the years or even decades that some people continue using them.

Why do people keep taking sleeping pills if the pills no longer work? The reason is *rebound insomnia*.

Rebound Insomnia

Once your body has learned to rely on pills for sleep, taking the pills away may cause your insomnia to be much worse than if you'd never taken any pills. This is called rebound insomnia. Sometimes, rebound insomnia can go on for several weeks.

Taking sleeping pills is like borrowing money from the bank. For awhile, you can "borrow" sleep by using pills. But eventually, you have to "pay back" the sleep—with insomnia. There is no other pill, no magic wand, that can save you from this payback. You can't escape rebound insomnia by taking one kind of sleeping pill one week and another kind the next. They are all cross-tolerant and will have the same effect as if you'd stuck with just one kind of pill. Occasionally, borrowing may be useful—but when you do, be sure you are ready to pay it back at a later time.

Sleeping Pills Can Cause Addiction

Because of rebound insomnia, you can become addicted to sleeping pills. Although the pills don't actually help you sleep anymore, you keep taking them—because if you don't, you'll have insomnia that is worse than what you had before you started taking the pills.

Once you start using sleeping pills, there is always a chance that you might get dependent on them. This is why many sleep experts are against ever using pills to sleep. Before you start, ask yourself if you will have the courage and strength to take them only occasionally. If you doubt yourself, ask your physician to prescribe only a very few pills at a time.

There are people who form addictions to almost anything. If they take a painkiller, they become addicted to it; if they drink alcohol, they become alcoholics; if they gamble, they become gambling addicts. And if they take sleeping pills, they get hooked on them. If you've had previous experiences where things took over your life—alcohol, smoking, overeating—you must be very careful. It's better to do without sleeping pills entirely than to get addicted to them.

T. R. Dutch, a 62-year-old small-business owner, was referred to the Dartmouth Sleep Disorders Center in 1976. He slept very little or not at all, even though he regularly took at least 40 mg of Valium, 90 mg of Dalmane, and 400 mg of Seconal each night! (These are extremely high dosages.) When this mixture did not induce sleep, he often consumed up to a fifth of whiskey as well.

T. R. had been referred to the sleep clinic after a severe blackout; such blackouts sometimes occurred, he said, after he took "whole handfuls" of sleeping pills. Four times in the past, his wife had found him unconscious on the floor and was unable to arouse him. On one occasion, he had remained comatose for five days!

In the sleep laboratory, his usual nightly dose of sleeping pills produced no normal sleep. Although the EEG slowed somewhat for about two hours toward morning (indicating that he was dozing), nothing in the EEG record resembled normal sleep. Nevertheless, T. R. claimed that his laboratory sleep was much better than usual.

We could hardly believe what we found when we took his history. He'd been a good sleeper until two weeks after Pearl Harbor, when he'd been appointed manager of the plant where he worked after most of the other men joined the Army. Being ill prepared, he worried and slept poorly, and a barbiturate was prescribed. Thirty-five years later, he was still taking sleeping pills every night!

After he was admitted to an inpatient unit, T. R. was gradually withdrawn from all pills. He learned biofeedback and relaxation exercises, went to Alcoholics Anonymous for help with his drinking problem, and reestablished social ties with family and friends. A low-grade chronic depression was treated with an antidepressant and, within six months, he was functioning again. Four years later, he still slept only three to five hours a night, but arose more refreshed. He now uses sleeping pills only rarely, if he's had two or three extremely poor nights in a row, and even then in much lower dosages.

Don't get into the same trouble as T. R. Dutch did. Eventually, you'll have to pay back the sleep you borrowed.

Sleeping Pills Can Mask Other Problems

A sleeping pill can be masking the real causes of poor sleep—the medical, behavioral, or psychological problems we have talked about—

and may be delaying treatment that could be curing the insomnia instead of just holding it down. We are in full agreement with the recommendations of the National Institutes of Health conference on insomnia: The treatment of insomnia should start with the correction of sleep hygiene and poor sleep habits before sleeping medication is used. After that, if pills must be used, then "Patients should receive the smallest effective dose for the shortest clinically necessary period of time."

A sleeping pill also can be used to hide a problem of boredom, especially in older people. Sleep is sometimes sought as an escape by very bored people when time hangs heavily on their hands. Life is so boring that they escape by going to bed. Insomnia develops from staying in bed too long, and the push for sleeping pills is on.

One especially frightening case occurred during research in our lab on a new sleeping pill that was being studied to determine the recommended dosage for the elderly. Anna Park was an 85-year-old widow, a friendly, quiet woman who couldn't sleep and who came to the sleep lab every night for ten nights as part of the research program. She was driven home by a taxi driver every morning and brought back to the lab every evening. Each night, when asked about any side effects, Mrs. Park said, "Lovely, the pills are just lovely. I sleep so soundly. There are no side effects." This went on for six days.

On the evening of the seventh day, the taxi driver called in a panic: "I'm at her house—she didn't answer the doorbell, so I went in, and she's lying on the couch, out cold." He was told to bring her in right away. We had emergency preparations ready and immediately monitored her brain waves and heart rate. We found deep sleep, nothing else wrong with her. The emergency team decided it was safest for her to sleep right in the lab where we could watch her all night.

The next morning, Mrs. Park woke up, and we asked what happened. "Doctor, those are the best sleeping pills." "But we found you on the couch and nobody could wake you up!" "Well, that's what's so great about these pills. I not only sleep in the lab, I sleep in the taxi home, and I sleep all day at home." She had gotten a heavy overdose, but she thought the effects were fantastic. She barely had to face life at all. She slept most of the day and most of the night, and that was her goal.

Older people need stimulation during the day to sleep well at night. The family can play a role: Bring things to older relatives to

make life less boring, have the kids stop in after school for ten minutes—
do anything to help make life more interesting. Nursing homes can
offer more stimulating activities, allow residents to have more personal
belongings and hobby materials, and allow radios, stereos, and tele-
phones in their rooms.

Sleeping Pills Can Affect the Day After

People usually take sleeping pills for one of two reasons: to try to
sleep better at night, or because they hope to improve alertness the
next day. Pills may help you sleep somewhat better, but research shows
that they do not improve mental or motor performance on the following day.

When performance tasks such as driving simulations were assessed
after nights on pills and nights on placebo, the pills often impaired
performance the next day even more than a night of poor sleep.
Insomnia can leave a person groggy and sleepy, but sleeping pills can
do the same thing, sometimes worse.

Dozens of studies have backed up these results. Whether people
were asked to add numbers, play video games, copy drawings, make
decisions, or remember words, their performance was never better
after a night of sleeping well with a pill than after a night of sleeping
poorly with a placebo. A typical study done by researchers at the
Naval Health Research Center of San Diego, for example, showed that
in *no case* did people who took sleeping pills handle tasks better the
next day than they did when not taking pills.

The reason is that a portion of the sleeping medication typically
remains in the body much longer than the few hours for which it was
taken to aid sleep, making you sedated and groggy the next day. This
hangover effect is worst with sleeping pills that are metabolized very
slowly, such as Dalmane.

The best that can be said about the sleeping pills currently available
is that after using them for a night, your performance may be as good
as if you hadn't taken a pill at all. And this can be said only for pills
that are metabolized fast, such as Halcion. If you are afraid of those
long, sleepless nights, a pill may help you sleep, but it is a myth that
it will help you function better the next day.

Sleeping Pills Can Cause Side Effects

According to *Physician's Drug Alert* (July 1988), a single high dose of the sleeping pill Halcion was reported to have caused short term amnesia in five hospitalized elderly people. Another report on this drug revealed that it had caused temporary amnesia in three middle-aged men who had taken it to try to minimize the effects of jet lag. While these pills are safe when taken occasionally in low dosages, high dosages can get you into trouble.

The scary part about it is that people do not feel confused in any way and are not aware that their memory is impaired. They function well, but later they simply do not remember what they did. One professor gave a lecture; later that day, when a student came up to him and asked a question about one of the topics, he didn't even remember giving the lecture!

To put these things into perspective, massive memory losses have occurred only with *very* high dosages of Halcion. To our knowledge, they have *never* happened when Halcion was given in the currently recommended dosages of 0.125 mg or 0.25 mg. We are telling these stories not to scare you off Halcion, but to warn you against impulsive doubling or redoubling any sleeping pill if the single dose does not work. Check with your doctor before you increase the dosage of any medication.

All sleeping pills have been shown to have side effects. They may cause high blood pressure, anxiety, dizziness, weakness, restlessness, nausea, confusion, poor coordination, delayed reaction time, digestive upset, loss of appetite, blurred vision, skin rash, and frequent urination.

Sleeping pills also slow down respiration. This doesn't usually make much difference unless you have a weak respiratory system or sleep apnea. When you take a sleeping pill, you breathe more slowly and more shallowly. When the respiratory center is slowed down, apneas that were 10 to 15 seconds long may become 40 seconds long, which drops the oxygen saturation in the blood to a low enough level to wake you up all night long. That is one reason that some people say, "I sleep worse with sleeping pills than without."

If you have serious sleep apnea, the risk from taking a sleeping pill is quite frightening. One case was reported of a 72-year-old man with severe sleep apnea who, in a research study, took a standard dose of a popular sleeping pill. His apneas usually lasted about 45 seconds when he was not on a sleeping pill. The night he took the sleeping pill, the pauses in breathing lasted three minutes! One episode even lasted five minutes—so long that the researcher feared for the man's life and awakened him. Serious sleep apnea and sleeping pills simply don't mix.

This aggravation of apnea with sleeping pills can occur in middle-aged people, too. Dr. Wallace Mendelson of Stony Brook, New York, reported a case of a 38-year-old man who had 2 to 18 apneas on no-pill nights—not considered anything to worry about—but had 100 apneas on the second night on a sleeping pill.

Because of all these possible side effects, we urge that you always take the lowest possible dosage of a sleeping pill. Many people do not need the full dosage. Find out for yourself if you do. Tell your doctor you would like to try taking only half the usual prescribed dosage. If it works, great! If not, you can always go onto the full dosage the next night. But *never* increase dosages or take more pills than your doctor has prescribed. You could do serious damage.

The stories of side effects in nursing-home patients make sad reading. Because of the excessive use of sleeping pills and other sedating drugs, people in some nursing homes often plod through the day lethargic and tired or even in a drugged daze. And because the pills can cause lack of coordination, there are unnecessary accidents and falls. Sometimes, for example, an older person who needs to get up in the middle of the night to go to the bathroom may stumble and fall, even breaking a hip, because he or she is disoriented from a heavy dose of sleeping pills. Sometimes there is memory loss, confusion, and even delirium.

An article in the *Journal of the American Medical Association* states that both sedatives and sleeping pills are still overly and improperly used in nursing homes. In a study reported in the *American Journal of Psychiatry* (November 1988), Drs. Michael G. Moran, Troy L. Thompson II, and Alan Nies found that 20 percent of patients studied in nursing homes lacked coordination or developed hallucinations because of sleeping pills. Dr. Mark Beers, now at UCLA, and colleagues at the Harvard Medical School in Boston studied residents of 12 nursing homes in Massachusetts and also found heavy use of high levels of sedatives, sleeping pills, and antipsychotic drugs. The pills often were given on a scheduled basis, rather than as needed. The drugs were not prescribed for special need, the authors said, but were used as a "chemical restraint."

Ray Rothman is a dramatic example of what can happen. He had been happily married for 43 years, but with increasing age, he developed leg problems and had to use a wheelchair. As he became increasingly infirm, his elderly wife was no longer able to take care of him. His family reluctantly decided to put him into a nursing home. Mr. Rothman fought the decision, claiming that he was able to take care of himself. He was a difficult patient in the nursing home, bent on escape. On many occasions, he got as far as the lobby or even out into the street, where he tried to wheel his chair into the driving lane to make motorists stop and take him home.

The nursing staff then tied his wheelchair to his bed to prevent further escapes. Mr. Rothman gave up and spent most of his day lying in bed dozing. As a result, he was often awake at night, rummaging through the home, causing commotion, making noise, and, at least twice, trying to escape again. The lone nighttime nurse on duty could not handle him in addition to the 40 other patients who were in the home, and the physician on duty reluctantly prescribed sleeping pills to keep Mr. Rothman quiet at night. However, because Mr. Rothman also slept during the day, the doctor had to prescribe relatively high dosages to keep him sedated.

Although Mr. Rothman was now more manageable, he often was confused. When his family came for visits, especially when they awakened him from a dream, he often was disoriented, thinking he was back in his childhood, or unable to distinguish his dreams from reality. In his confusion, he accused others of abusing him, felt that the staff was trying to rob him, demanded to know why he was incarcerated, and became very irrational. To counteract this, an antipsychotic medication was prescribed. The combination of sedatives and antipsychotics caused Mr. Rothman to become even less coordinated and coherent. One night, he attempted to go to the bathroom, fell, and broke his hip. He could not understand the cast and felt that it was a straitjacket that had been put on him as part of his undeserved incarceration.

Luckily, at this time, a new physician arrived, better trained in geriatric medicine. He tapered the medication, and Mr. Rothman's mind cleared dramatically. He encouraged the staff to interact with Mr. Rothman, keeping him awake during the day talking about old

memories, and he encouraged Mr. Rothman's children to take their
father out for occasional drives. Once he was even allowed to go home
and visit with his wife in the old apartment. Although he never lost
his desire to return home, he understood much better what was happening, and the nightmare that had started with an inappropriate
prescription of sleeping pills lightened considerably.

The routine use of sleeping pills in many nursing homes is partly
a staffing problem. There is limited nursing staff at night, so the decision sometimes is made to sedate patients at night. There are fewer
nursing homes that do it now than there were 20 years ago, but it still
occurs and needs to be watched for.

The use of sleeping pills in hospitals also is decreasing. Most
doctors now write orders that sleeping pills should be given only if
the patient requests one or if the nurse feels the patient needs one.
But routine administration still occurs. We all know the joke about
the nurse waking up the hospital patient because it's time for a sleeping
pill. It happens less now, but it still happens.

Not only can sleeping pills make hospital patients groggy the next
day, but they also can interact with other medications and possibly
affect test results. Worst of all, patients may have been started on a
long term dependency on sleeping pills—when they never needed
them in the first place.

If You Are Pregnant

Most people have heard about thalidomide, the once widely used
sedative that produced birth defects in many babies. Preliminary research indicates that some other sleeping pills, in rare cases, also might
cause deformities of the fetus, especially if a pregnant woman takes
them in the first trimester.

Another problem: If a mother is addicted to sleeping pills, her
newborn infant may undergo the same kind of withdrawal symptoms
that an adult would: irritability, insomnia, tremors, and hyperactivity.

No drug has been proven completely safe for a fetus and sleeping
pills are no exception. Do not take sleeping pills if you are pregnant
or if there is even a possibility of your being pregnant—that is, if you
are a woman of child-bearing age and not using efficient methods of
birth control.

Remember, too, that if you're breast-feeding your child, sleeping medications can be transferred through your milk and cause problems in the infant.

Sleeping Pills Can Cause Accidents

Because reaction time and thinking are slowed by sleeping pills, their use can be disastrous for people driving automobiles or operating heavy or dangerous machinery. Studies in both Finland and Great Britain show that persons taking sleeping pills had a higher incidence of automobile accidents than did others.

On the day after taking a sleeping pill, you may have a hangover effect slowing you down. You may feel alert, even though you're not. So do not take a sleeping pill that causes daytime sedation if, early the next day, you need to drive more than a short distance or do other tasks that are potentially dangerous.

Sleeping Pills Can Interact with Other Drugs

If you are taking other medications in addition to sleeping pills, the amount of any other drug you are taking may need to be adjusted. For example, Tagamet (prescribed for ulcers) is metabolized by the same liver enzymes that metabolize most sleeping pills. If you are taking such sleeping pills, your Tagamet level would be wrong and your doctor would need to adjust it.

All sleeping pills are central-nervous-system depressants. They slow down the activity in the nervous system, as do antihistamines and tranquilizers. If you take one of these plus a sleeping pill, your nervous system would be slowed down even more.

If sleeping pills are prescribed for you and you are taking other pills, be sure to remind your doctor of them, especially if they have been prescribed by another physician.

Sleeping Pills Plus Alcohol Can Kill You

Most people do not realize just how dangerous a sleeping-pill-and-alcohol mix can be. Each adds to the effects of the other. This is especially true for respiration; each drug by itself slows respiration, and together they can cause serious problems.

It is frightening just how often people still combine the two. Sometimes, an insomniac person will take a few drinks to help relax and then later take a high dose of a sleeping pill, never realizing the danger. In some cases, even one glass of wine or liquor could be dangerous; so you should simply *never* drink alcohol when you have taken, or are about to take, a sleeping pill.

The newer kinds of sleeping pills are not as dangerous as older kinds, but there still is the danger of an accidental, or even suicidal, overdose, especially if the pills are mixed with alcohol or other drugs. Sleeping pills have been involved in the deaths of many well-known people, such as Dorothy Kilgallen, Marilyn Monroe, and, recently, the radical activist Abbie Hoffman.

All Sleeping Pills Are Not Alike

Some sleeping pills act quickly, while others have a lag time before they act. Some act for only a few hours, others may last into the next day. All of these factors are important if and when you and your doctor decide that you need a sleeping pill.

Some pills, such as Dalmane and Halcion, are fast in uptake, so you should take them when you go to bed; Restoril and others are slow in uptake, so you should take them half an hour before going to bed. (*Uptake* refers to how fast after you take a sleeping pill the chemical is in your brain working.) If you ever have to take a pill in the middle of the night, you also would want a fast-uptake pill.

Also important is *half-life*—the time it takes for your body to break down and eliminate half the drug that you took. Halcion has a quick half-life of five hours (after five hours, half of it is gone). Because your body gets rid of it fast, it has less effect on the next day's performance. One of the longest acting sleeping pills is Dalmane. It affects daytime performance considerably and, if you take it for more than one night, the effect can be additive and you can be sleepy for days.

There is quite a bit of argument among sleep experts about whether a long-acting or a short-acting pill is better. Some believe that you should use long-acting pills if you are upset and want to have some daytime sedation as well. Then, instead of taking a sleeping pill at night and a tranquilizer during the day, you could take only a long-acting sleeping pill that would have some carryover of sedation the next day. If you need to be alert and active during the day, pills with shorter half-lives are better.

Older patients, who tend to clear drugs from their systems more slowly, are more likely to develop mental and motor impairments when given long-acting pills. Poor coordination and problems with memory and thinking are possible complications. Similar problems may develop in younger patients who have impaired kidney or liver function, such as some alcoholics.

The ideal sleeping pill would have just enough accumulation in the blood to work, would cause no side effects, and would cause no performance loss or hangover on the following morning. Unfortunately, no sleeping pill like this exists.

The Kinds of Sleeping Pills

Benzodiazepines

The benzodiazepines currently are the sleeping pills of choice in most situations. They are marketed also as tranquilizers and muscle relaxants. The benzodiazepines also include the tranquilizers Valium, Librium, and Ativan, as well as Dalmane, Restoril, and Halcion.

These drugs are the safest of the sleeping pills and are the least likely to cause side effects. However, you still can build up a dependence on them, they still can depress breathing just like all the other sleeping pills, you still get rebound insomnia when you stop taking them, and they still can cause death when taken in combination with alcohol. Also, in large doses, all benzodiazepines are known to have detrimental effects on memory.

FLURAZEPAM (DALMANE)

Flurazepam is absorbed rapidly; its half-life is about 8 to 12 hours. Unfortunately, however, some of it is metabolized into another chemical that also induces sleep and has an elimination half-life that ranges from 50 to 300 hours, depending on the status of the patient's liver functions. Because of this, taking flurazepam causes daytime sedation. It also has been incriminated in several episodes of depression, irritability, and temper outbursts.

For most patients, the 15-mg dosage is as effective as 30 mg, while causing fewer side effects.

TEMAZEPAM (RESTORIL)

Temazepam has a slower absorption rate than many other benzodiazepines and a half-life of about eight hours. It should be given one-half hour before bedtime. Thus, it is useful if you know ahead of time that you want to take a sleeping pill. It is *not* useful when you want a sleeping pill in the middle of the night.

TRIAZOLAM (HALCION)

Triazolam has a fast absorption rate and an elimination half-life of about five hours. This medication is preferred if daytime sedation needs to be avoided (while flurazepam is preferred if such sedation is desired). In fact, there appears to be an increase in daytime alertness in patients taking triazolam at bedtime. This is considered an advantage by some physicians, but others worry about rebound anxiety. We consider it safe up to 0.25 mg, but advise against higher dosages.

Barbiturates

The barbiturates were the sleeping pills of choice in the early 20th century. The early barbiturates were so long-lasting that those who took them were sleepy all night and all day. Later, shorter-acting barbiturates were created. Barbiturates are used less today, but occasionally the benzodiazepines are not effective, and a barbiturate is used. However, barbiturate overdoses are much more dangerous than overdoses of benzodiazepines. Barbiturates have more side effects, are more rapidly addictive, and may produce frequent awakenings and disturbing dreams. People often develop tolerance to barbiturates quickly, become dependent on them, and then may be tempted to increase the dosage without asking their doctor, little realizing how dangerous this can be. The combination of barbiturates and alcohol can be fatal. Barbiturates also interact more with other drugs.

The barbiturates include secobarbital (Seconal), amobarbital (Amytal), pentobarbital (Nembutal), and a combination of secobarbital and amobarbital (Tuinal). They have half-lives of 14 to 48 hours.

Chloral Hydrate

Chloral hydrate, an older sleeping pill, may be useful in patients who cannot take benzodiazepines or barbiturates. The problem is that it has serious side effects in high dosages, so chloral hydrate should be used only in special situations or in a hospital setting where side effects can be carefully watched for. (It was chloral hydrate that, mixed in a cocktail, produced the famous Mickey Finn knockout.)

Antihistamines

When antihistamines are given for allergies, drowsiness is an unwanted side effect. For the insomniac, the side effect is the reason for taking the pill.

Sleep experts are not impressed by antihistamines. True, 100 mg of Benadryl may be a mild sleeping pill, but its side effects are worse than those of a similarly effective, tiny dose of a benzodiazepine.

Antidepressants

Although more research is needed, very low dosages of tricyclic antidepressants (such as 25 mg of Elavil) seem to induce sleep quite well in certain patients, especially those with childhood-onset insomnia and those with nonrestorative sleep. In fact, the tricyclics seem to be less habit-forming when given as sleeping pills than are the benzodiazepines.

So if your doctor wants you to try a very low dosage of an antidepressant, it's not necessarily because he or she thinks you're depressed, but because some antidepressants help you sleep. However, they have their own side effects, even in low dosages. They can, for example, cause dry mouth, constipation, fast pulse, urinary problems, or impotence.

Tranquilizers

Tranquilizers were designed to aid relaxation and relieve anxiety. They also can be used as sleeping pills.

They are relatively safe when taken in small doses, but can be addictive. Taking too high a dosage can cause confusion, impaired judgment, drowsiness, irritability, and motor disturbance.

Actually, tranquilizers and sleeping pills are basically the same thing. A tranquilizer given in a higher dosage will act as a sleeping pill, and a sleeping pill in a lower dosage can act as a daytime tranquilizer. The distinction often is made on the basis of marketing. You can't advertise a drug until you can prove that it works—and that is expensive. So Valium, for example, never has been adequately tested as a sleeping pill because it would cost considerable extra money to research that aspect of the drug. And Dalmane never has been tested as a tranquilizer. In practice, physicians often do use Valium as a sleeping pill.

Over-the-Counter (OTC) Sleep Aids

These include such pills as Sleep-Eze, Nytol, and Sominex. They make you groggy and drowsy, which sometimes can help you fall asleep. They may be useful if you are worrying about sleep or if you are trying too hard to sleep.

The OTCs have the same problem as prescription pills: If you take them night after night, they won't work any more. So don't take one the first night of poor sleep, but only if you have had poor sleep for several nights in a row and you are getting worried about it or it starts affecting your job.

OTC medications advertised as sleeping pills usually contain antihistamines. (Until recently, they sometimes contained pyrilamine, scopolamine, and bromides, but these were just banned by the FDA as being of unproven effectiveness.) Although the amounts of antihistamine used are low, there still are possible side effects if you are sensitive to them.

The ingredients in OTC sleeping pills change so often that the only way you can be sure of the current composition is to go to the drugstore and read the most recent label. The names may be the same, but what is in them changes frequently.

Aspirin

· • • ● • • ·

When I was at Dartmouth, so many insomniacs told me that aspirin worked as a sleeping pill that my colleague, Dr. Peter M. Silberfarb, and I tested it. Eight men and women who had had serious insomnia for at least two years volunteered for the study. On some nights, a pla-

cebo pill was given; on other nights, two aspirins (650 mg) were given. Six of the eight patients had better sleep with aspirin.

The surprising finding was that there was about a four-hour delay in its effect. We gave it at bedtime, and it had its effect not so much on going to sleep as during the second half of the night. The aspirin seemed to result in relatively normal sleep, since none of the sleep stages were disturbed, and there was no hangover the following day.

So if waking up frequently in the middle of the night is a problem, you might try using aspirin at bedtime instead of a sleeping pill. Take two aspirins just before bedtime with a full glass of water. But this seems to be effective for only a few nights, so take it not more than twice per week.

You should not take aspirin, however, if you have an ulcer or other intestinal disorders or a tendency for bleeding, since aspirin tends to thin the blood.

· · ● ● · · ·

How to Kick the Habit

As we have said before, if you have been taking sleep medication and then stop abruptly, you usually will suffer from insomnia for at least a few nights, occasionally for weeks. Ironically, this rebound insomnia usually is worse than the insomnia you had before you started the pills. It appears that the higher the dosage, the longer you will have the withdrawal symptoms. (Remember that you can never buy sleep, you can only borrow it—later on, you have to pay it back.)

As part of withdrawal, you may have serious trouble getting to sleep or you may wake up often in the middle of the night. More rarely, you may have nightmares. If you have been taking drugs that are suppressants of REM sleep (for example, antidepressants), you may experience *REM rebound*—too much dreaming and, possibly, frequent awakening from nightmares.

It is important not to go back on the pills again. This just perpetuates the problem. The rebound insomnia and nightmares are only temporary. Often, the first night is the worst.

Other withdrawal symptoms, if you withdraw cold turkey, may include fatigue, weakness, depression, jitteriness, shakiness, changes in taste and smell, cramps, nausea, headache, and even convulsions (if you withdraw from high doses of barbiturates). That's why we recommend *gradual* withdrawal if you have been on sleeping pills for a long time.

Here are the steps you should take if you now use sleeping pills and have decided to stop:

1. Get very competent with relaxation techniques and the other parts of our program. In other words, polish your nondrug weapons for fighting insomnia to give yourself extra help.
2. Pick a specific time to quit, giving yourself at least four weeks for withdrawal. Some people pick a vacation as a nonstress time. Others figure they wouldn't sleep during stress anyway, so they might as well go through withdrawal during a stressful time and get it over with.
3. Announce your plan to others. Talk about the anticipated "last day of pill bondage." Having announced your plan to all who care will help you stick to it later.
4. Make a specific withdrawal plan. Keep only the medication that you plan to need to get through your withdrawal period. Give the excess to a trusted friend. The first week, cut down by one-fourth the dosage that you now take. Each week after that, cut down to half of what you took the week before, until you are down to just a little dust on the last week. (Cut a tablet with a sharp knife. If the pills come in capsule form, open the capsule and remove some of the contents. Each week remove more until you get down to nothing.) If you have difficulties with this plan, take smaller steps and stretch your withdrawal over six or eight weeks; but whatever step you have reached, don't go backward.
5. Have a supply of books or materials for some favorite hobby handy to use during the possible nights of sleeplessness. Continue your exercise, relaxation training, and social life. Think about how much better your sleep is going to be and how much better you will feel in the daytime from now on.
6. On the day of the last pill, have a celebration. At whatever celebration you choose, flush away all the leftover pills.

If withdrawal by yourself is too difficult, you may have to work with a doctor or other professional, or even spend a week or so in a hospital where you can get medical and counseling support. Indeed, withdrawing from heavy use of sleeping pills is sometimes more difficult than withdrawing from heroin; in some cases, patients have had to be admitted to our alcohol and drug-addiction unit for up to four weeks before they succeeded in becoming pill-free.

Occasional Use of Sleeping Pills

There is no question that natural sleep is the best, but there are times—for example, in periods of grief or pain or after surgery—when pills to aid sleep may be of benefit.

Louise Ludlow was an emotional, high-strung person and physically not very healthy. She always had stomach problems, often to the point of having to be fed artificially because she could not keep food down. Now she was going to be married, and she couldn't sleep at all. It was five days before the wedding, she was getting circles under her eyes, and she couldn't function. She came to the clinic, crying. We advised her: "Take the pills for the few nights before the wedding if you want, but you will pay with some nights of insomnia afterward. So after the wedding, know that you will have several poor nights of sleep." The pills helped to get her through.

Most sleep experts consider it acceptable to use a pill occasionally. If, for example, you haven't slept for two or three nights, or it's 1 A.M. and you're tossing and turning, wide awake from worry, and tomorrow you have to be extra sharp for an important event, it sometimes can be of benefit to take a pill. But before you do it, make a contract with yourself that you are not going to take any more pills that week—limit yourself to a maximum of one pill a week.

It is okay, in our judgment, to have in your medicine cabinet a *few* sleeping pills (*not* 50 or 100). Just knowing that a few pills are available, even if you don't use them, sometimes can ease worries and help you sleep.

If You Decide to Use a Sleeping Pill

Summary: There are only two situations in which sleeping pills are possibly indicated:

1. You are going through an acute, short term crisis and you cannot handle it without sleeping pills

2. You have chronic serious insomnia, and you want to borrow some sleep with a pill every so often to get adequate rest

If you have decided that you are in a situation where you really would be helped by a sleeping pill, here is a summary of guidelines to follow in taking it:

- Buy the lowest dosage form of the pill, then use half a pill to see if it will work. Always use the lowest possible dosage that works for you, especially after age 60.
- Be sure you have no medical condition that can be worsened by the pills. If you have liver or kidney disease, discuss with your doctor whether you should have a lower dosage or not take pills at all.
- Never take a higher dosage than your doctor has recommended, even if you still have trouble falling asleep or if you awaken in the middle of the night. Never increase the dosage if the old dosage doesn't work any more. Should effectiveness diminish, discontinue the pill for a month or two and it will help again.
- Take the pill according to its uptake time, as discussed earlier, depending on when and how long you want it to work.
- If you are taking any other drugs, be sure to tell your doctor, since sleeping pills can interact with other drugs, even if the sleeping pills are nonprescription, over-the-counter.
- If pain is causing you to have poor sleep, ask for a painkiller, not a sleeping pill. If you are depressed, discuss with your doctor taking an antidepressant instead of a sleeping pill.
- Do not take a pill after midnight, because it may give you a pill hangover the next day.
- After you have taken a pill, do not drive or use dangerous machinery.
- If you feel dizzy, unsteady, less alert, or sleepy during the day after using a sleeping pill, discuss with your doctor changing the dosage or changing to a different pill.
- *Do not consume alcohol if you take a sleeping pill*—the combination can cause serious complications, even death.
- Use the pills only for short term management and never get a standing order for sleeping pills or automatic refills without discussing it with your doctor. As soon as the short term crisis is over, get off the pill immediately.

- Remember that each time you take a pill, you will have to pay back your borrowed sleep later on.

When You Should Not Use Sleeping Pills

- Never give sleeping pills to a child.
- Never use sleeping pills if you are pregnant, or think you could become pregnant.
- Do not use sleeping pills if you ever have had problems with addictions of any kind (alcohol, drugs, gambling).
- Never use sleeping pills if you are a habitual loud snorer or have been told that you seem to have difficulty breathing when you sleep. Go to a sleep center to determine if you have sleep apnea.
- Whenever possible, instead of taking a pill, do all the other things that have been discussed in this book. Hopefully, if you follow our program, you won't need pills—because you will have found other, better ways to solve insomnia.

···•· 15 ·•···

Other Sleep Disorders

There are other sleep disorders in addition to insomnia. Although we are not discussing them as extensively as we do insomnia, it is good to know a little about them, because they often are interrelated with insomnia and even sometimes mimic insomnia, causing symptoms that can be confused with it.

These sleep disorders generally fall into two categories: excessive daytime sleepiness and parasomnias. We will discuss both types in this chapter. We'll also talk about a few disorders that don't fit in either category.

Excessive Daytime Sleepiness

A woman wrote to *Dear Abby* and asked about her boyfriend who, she said, kept falling asleep in the most unusual circumstances. "You can't imagine how I feel when we are talking or making love, and suddenly he's out like a light".

Abby suggested that she have her friend see a physician, the sooner the better. Abby was right. Although we have stressed self-help in this book, there are some conditions that need medical attention, and excessive daytime sleepiness is one of them.

If you have this disorder of excessive daytime sleepiness, you are extremely sleepy during the day even though your nighttime sleep seems to be adequate. You're not just tired or depressed or bored, it's not just fatigue—you actually fall asleep in situations when others would not. For example, we know of a factory worker who was called for a disciplinary hearing because he often fell asleep on the job. While the boss was furiously yelling at him about his laziness, the man fell asleep! We also know of a widower who had two teenage daughters he was raising. When they misbehaved and he became angry at them, he would suddenly fall asleep. When he woke up, his daughters would be nowhere to be found.

How can you tell whether you are just tired or depressed, or actually have true excessive daytime sleepiness that you should be concerned about? A depressed person typically will say something like: "If only I could take a nap, I would feel better, but I can't. I don't feel sleepy. I'm just tired all the time. I don't have any ambition, my mind wanders—but I can't fall asleep." In contrast, a person who has excessive daytime sleepiness *does* fall asleep during the day. In response to the same question, he or she may say, "Usually I can't even watch a TV show or a movie or write or sew without dozing off. Sometimes I fall asleep in my car when I am waiting for a light to change. I may even fall asleep at parties or in the middle of a conversation."

There is a procedure called the *multiple sleep latency test* (MSLT) that we use to assess how sleepy a person is. Patients sleep in the lab for one night to make sure that they have a full night's sleep; then, during the day, they are asked to lie down every two hours for 20 minutes, and technicians measure whether and how fast they fall asleep. An alert person might fall asleep once during the four nap times, say after lunch. A diagnosis of excessive sleepiness is made if the patient falls asleep on each of the four nap times in an average of five minutes or less. (People without this problem wouldn't fall asleep each time in five minutes or less unless they had not slept at all for 48 hours.)

You can do an at-home version of the MSLT to help test for excessive daytime sleepiness. First, get a good night's sleep. Then, lie down every two hours throughout the day, say at 9 A.M., 11 A.M., 1 P.M., and 3 P.M. Hold a set of keys in two fingers over the side of the bed when you lie down. When you fall asleep, the keys will drop, and the noise they make will wake you up. If the keys drop, on the average, in less than five minutes during these tests, you have pretty good evidence that you are excessively sleepy.

If you are excessively sleepy, our first advice is to try for a week to sleep at least one or even two hours longer. A frequent problem with excessively sleepy people is that they simply do not give themselves enough time to sleep. You may simply be staying up too late, or you may be an extra-long sleeper, needing nine to ten hours of sleep before you feel refreshed. If the increased time in bed for a week makes you less sleepy, then you simply need to make room in your schedule for more sleep.

Dr. Howard R. Roffwarg, of the University of Texas Medical Center in Dallas, tells the story of a Puerto Rican hospital attendant he knew many years ago who was extremely sleepy throughout the day and finally sought help. Juan was quite concerned about his health and had no idea what was wrong. He fell asleep right in the middle of the interview. Careful questioning revealed the reason: As is typical of his culture, the man stayed up every night until 1 or 2 A.M. However, having a hospital job, he had to get up at 5 A.M., and he couldn't take the traditional siesta. So he was simply sleep-deprived.

If increased time in bed does not help and you still are excessively sleepy, you should be seen at a sleep disorders center. It is likely that a medical condition is causing your problem, and things can be done to help. People sometimes are ridiculed for years because they fall asleep all the time, or they may be called lazy or stupid. The truth is that these disorders are almost never caused by a psychiatric or psychological problem. It usually is a medical condition such as sleep apnea, narcolepsy, twitching movements of the legs during sleep, or other medical problem such as an infection, a neurological disorder, or withdrawal from certain drugs.

There are four simple questions to ask that can help with the diagnosis of what causes excessive daytime sleepiness:

1. Do you snore loudly or appear to stop breathing during the night? Ask your bed partner. If so, you may have sleep apnea.
2. Do you ever suddenly become weak all over and need to sit down? If this happens, especially when you are excited, angry, or upset, and you are under age 35, you may have narcolepsy.
3. Do your legs twitch and kick repeatedly during the night? Again, ask your bed partner. If so, you may have a condition called periodic limb movements (previously called nocturnal myoclonus).
4. Have you recently started taking a medication, or recently withdrawn from one? Many medications can cause extreme sleepiness. And stopping stimulants, sleeping pills, tranquilizers, alcohol, or even caffeine also can cause drowsiness and the need for frequent napping.

If you answered yes to any of these questions, you should discuss the situation with your physician. If a drug is involved, you may need to be switched to a different dosage or to an alternative medication without sleep side effects. If you have apnea, narcolepsy, or periodic limb movements, you will want to be referred to a sleep disorders center.

By the way, if your doctor starts talking about "DIMS" and "DOES," he or she has not picked up a Brooklyn accent, but is referring to the two main types of sleep disorders: disorders of initiating and maintaining sleep (DIMS) and disorders of excessive somnolence (DOES) DIMS is simply a fancy term for insomnia. Your doctor also may talk about dyssomnia, which refers to either insomnia, disorders of excessive somnolence, or circadian rhythm problems.

Sleep Apnea

The term *apnea* means the absence of respiration. An episode of sleep apnea may last anywhere from ten seconds to two or three minutes. The person then awakens, may thrash around, gasps for air a few times, and falls asleep again. Another apnea usually begins again soon.

There are two types of apnea. In one type—*central apnea*—your respiratory center doesn't activate the drive to breathe and you awaken 10 to 60 seconds later for lack of air. This can happen for a few minutes at sleep onset, or it can go on throughout the entire night. In the other type—*obstructive sleep apnea*—when you fall asleep, the upper airway actually closes and you cannot move air, even though you try. This can be caused by anatomical problems such as, a very big uvula (the tissue that hangs down in the back of your throat), or a tongue that is set too far back in your mouth, so that it is sucked in when you breathe. In other cases, fat deposits narrow the airway. Occasionally, the airway simply is too small and flaccid and gets sucked shut when you breathe in.

People with serious sleep apnea typically complain about excessive daytime sleepiness. However, patients with milder forms may complain about insomnia, saying that they wake up repeatedly at night for unknown reasons.

Jerry Kern was an early case of sleep apnea seen at Dartmouth almost 20 years ago. He was a 45-year-old, severely obese (313 pounds), college-educated man who complained of always being sleepy during the day. His problems started when he was in his early 30s. Up to that time, he had been quite successful as a small businessman. After his early 30s, he never held any job for more than two or three weeks, and he usually got fired for "laziness," falling asleep five to ten times each day. For the 15 years before coming to the sleep lab, he had seen doctors all over the country and had spent more than $20,000 trying to find a cause for his sleepiness. However, except for gross obesity, high blood pressure, and some enlargement of the heart, none of his doctors could find anything abnormal.

Mr. Kern's personal life was in ruins—two wives had left him, preferring divorce to living with a chronically sleepy, obese snorer who couldn't hold a job. He couldn't maintain adequate social relationships with friends because of his continuing sleepiness, and he was flat broke.

In the lab, Mr. Kern was pleasant and polite. He fell asleep within 5 seconds after lights-out, but as soon as he fell asleep, his breathing stopped; then he woke up 35 seconds later gasping for air. This cycle repeated itself for the next 10 hours of "sleep." As soon as his EEG showed signs of sleep, his breathing stopped and he woke, gasping for air. Throughout the night, he never slept for more than three uninterrupted minutes. By morning, he had totaled 562 separate awakenings, and more than 75 percent of his "sleep" was spent not breathing!

In the morning, Mr. Kern was more tired than when he went to bed. He guessed that he had awakened "five to eight times" during the night, and he was totally unaware of his labored breathing, heavy snoring, and the more than 500 times he had stopped breathing.

He was told that he had sleep apnea, and various recommendations were made to him—including weight loss, which often helps. He declined to consider treatment for "a mere sleep problem."

The case had a sad ending. In the four months that followed, Mr. Kern became a heavy drinker, and a few months later he was caught in an armed robbery attempting to steal liquor. Eleven months after that, he died in his sleep in a state prison of "unknown causes."

Apnea can occur at all ages. However, the incidence increases dramatically with age. According to studies carried out in San Diego by Drs. Daniel Kripke and Sonia Ancoli-Israel, it is rare to find people over age 75 who do not show an occasional sleep apnea. Men outnumber women 30 to 1 in sleep apnea before menopause. After menopause, the ratio becomes more even. (Progesterone seems to be a respiratory stimulus that helps protect women from sleep apnea.)

An occasional apnea is quite common and is not significant. However, there is reason for concern if there are more than 15 to 20 apneas per hour or more than 100 per night—or if, together with the sleep apneas, a person complains about excessive daytime sleepiness. It is of special concern if the person has a heart condition, since it is difficult for the heart to beat when a person is desperately trying to move air and the air pressure in the lungs is not normal. Heart arrhythmias are common, and sometimes heart block occurs. In fact, there are many consequences of sleep apnea. Dr. Anthony Kales and his colleagues from Pennsylvania State University College of Medicine report that patients with apnea also may have morning headaches, high blood pressure, and cognitive impairment (can't think straight).

Apnea in children is especially tragic. Such children often are thought to be lazy, ummotivated, or dumb, when in reality they are simply sleepy from never sleeping enough at night. So if your child seems sleepy or lazy, listen at night to see if breathing is labored or there are pauses in breathing.

Sleep apnea in children often is caused by enlarged tonsils or adenoids. An occasional side effect from the many awakenings at night in children is bedwetting. A former colleague, Dr. Dudley Weider, from Dartmouth Medical School, observed that when he removed a child's tonsils, it sometimes cured the child's bedwetting. The sleep center team did a study and found that, indeed, such children often had sleep apnea.

TREATMENT

According to leading sleep researcher Dr. William Dement, 75 percent of the cases of sleep apnea are still undiagnosed. If you suspect that you have sleep apnea, you need to be evaluated in a sleep disorders center. There is no way around that. In the meantime:

Do not take sleeping pills.

Do not use alcohol.

Do not smoke.

Lose weight if you are overweight.

For temporary relief, try using many pillows, elevating the head of the bed, or sleeping in a recliner chair.

Avoid sleeping on your back. To help you, put a tennis ball in a sock and sew or pin it onto the back of your pajamas. (Dr. Rosalind Cartwright from the Rush-Presbyterian Medical Center in Chicago has a training program in which you wear a switch at night, and if you lie on your back, it sets off a loud whistle. Being awakened every time you lie on your back for a few days, you learn to avoid that position.)

Once you have been diagnosed, there are many treatment options.

Continuous positive airway pressure (CPAP) is currently the most used treatment. In this treatment, the patient attaches a mask to the nose before going to bed, and a small compressor delivers air at slightly above room pressure. This increased air pressure keeps the airways open, and the patient can breathe and sleep normally. Although it takes some getting used to, patients often are amazed at how much better they feel after only one or two nights with it.

Corrective surgery can be done if abnormalities in the upper airway are found. For example, if the tongue is set too far back, reconstructive jaw surgery might move it forward.

Occasionally, a procedure called UPPP (uvulopalatopharyngo-plasty) is recommended. This procedure acts like an internal facelift, tightening loose tissue. Patients often prefer surgery over CPAP because they don't have to be bothered by putting on a mask every night. However, UPPP is successful only about 50 percent of the time.

Tracheostomy is more drastic. A small hole is cut into the upper airway, and a special tube is inserted through the front of the neck. The tube is closed during the day; at night, the tube is opened to make breathing easier. This is an effective treatment, but it is hard to keep the tracheostomy clean, and sometimes it becomes infected or the opening gets covered with fibrous tissue.

Several drugs, including respiratory stimulants and progesterone, are being researched, but so far no drug has been found to be helpful in severe sleep apnea.

Another treatment that is reported to work in some cases is a tongue-retaining device that pulls the tongue forward so that it can't fall back into the throat. An appliance is fitted over the teeth with a bubble in front of the teeth. The patient sucks out the air and inserts the tongue, and the tongue is held forward for several hours. Other devices simply hold the lower jaw forward, which tends to open up the back of the airway.

SUPPORT GROUPS

For further information and location of a local network group of other sleep apnea patients, contact A.W.A.K.E., Association of Polysomnographic Technologists, Presbyterian University Hospital Sleep Evaluation Center, Pittsburgh, PA, 15213 (412–647–3464).

Narcolepsy

Buck Ulene was a 52-year-old married army officer referred to the sleep disorders center for evaluation of his excessive daytime sleepiness. He was sleepy throughout the day, even after good nights, and he had sleep attacks when the urge to sleep became so strong that he could not resist. He first experienced his sleepiness as an army recruit, and it was a continuing embarrassment, particularly when he fell asleep at meetings with his own officers. To compensate, he would hold a set of keys in his hand. If he went to sleep, the keys fell to the floor, the noise awakened him, and picking the keys up from the floor gave him some needed movement that made it possible to fight off sleep for another few minutes.

Several years later, he noticed that during periods of excitement or laughter, he sometimes would become very weak in his knees; occasionally, he collapsed and fell during these periods. His first episode occurred while fishing with his daughter: He caught a fish and then fell into the lake when he became weak from excitement. (Such periods of no muscle tone are called *cataplexy*.) The attacks became increasingly bothersome, until two or three episodes with nearly complete collapse occurred almost daily. As he got older, he learned to control his emotions, and as he became more stoic, the cataplectic attacks occurred less frequently.

Also, three or four times a week, he suddenly would feel unable to move while falling asleep. (This is called *sleep paralysis*.) At other times, again usually close to sleep onset, he vividly sensed the presence of other people in the room, occasionally even saw them or heard them, although he knew that he was alone. (These dream-like experiences just before falling asleep are called *hypnogogic hallucinations*.)

Mr. Ulene's physical and neurologic examinations showed nothing significant. But sleep in the lab was poor and riddled with many awakenings. The MSLT revealed an average sleep onset time of about two minutes, and REM (dreaming) periods usually occurred right at sleep onset. These findings indicated that Mr. Ulene was suffering from narcolepsy.

Mr. Ulene had considerable relief from a combination of stimulant and antidepressant medications. However, he gradually became tolerant of these drugs, and after many attempts to adjust the dosage, he finally was withdrawn from using them chronically. He now takes a stimulant only when needed, such as before long drives.

Mr. Ulene discussed his narcolepsy with his wife and with his commanding officers, who excused him from hazardous duties and allowed him to schedule two 20-minute naps each day. This provided considerable relief. Although he still experiences one or two episodes of cataplexy, sleep paralysis, or hypnogogic hallucinations per week, these episodes frighten him less now that he understands them.

In addition to excessive daytime sleepiness, cataplexy, hypnogogic hallucinations, and sleep paralysis, a person with narcolepsy sometimes also has *automatic behavior*—that is, the person behaves normally, but later does not remember extended periods of time. For example, a narcoleptic might suddenly find himself or herself ten exits farther down the freeway than he or she last remembered.

Paradoxically, narcoleptic patients often have poor nighttime sleep. We have had patients who thought that all their daytime symptoms were simply consequences of poor sleep—they came to the sleep lab requesting an evaluation of their insomnia, not their daytime sleepiness.

Narcolepsy typically starts between the ages of about 10 and 30. Symptoms are subtle at first and usually involve only excessive daytime sleepiness. The condition may remain mild, or it may progress, so that in a few years the person may fall asleep at a desk or in the middle of talking, eating, or making love. In extremely severe cases, the disease is so incapacitating that patients cannot hold jobs and are almost total invalids.

Narcolepsy is caused by physical, not psychological, factors, and the attacks have nothing to do with epilepsy, as is sometimes thought.

Estimates about the number of narcoleptic persons vary. A recent U.S. Department of Health report estimates the number at 100,000 to 250,000 cases in the United States. An American Medical Association publication estimates 400,000 to 600,000.

There clearly is a hereditary factor in narcolepsy. Close relatives of narcoleptics are 60 times more likely to be narcoleptic than is the general population, and narcolepsy recently has been the focus of several genetic studies that have yielded helpful results for understanding the disease.

TREATMENT

At present, there is no cure for narcolepsy, but several drugs are under development that look hopeful. Meanwhile, stimulants can help keep the patient alert, and antidepressants can suppress REM sleep, which helps to prevent cataplectic attacks. (One 80-year-old man with narcolepsy was most bothered when he played poker: When he got a good hand, the excitement set off a cataplectic attack, and everyone knew not to bet. He was not bothered at any other time, so he solved his problem by taking his medication before every poker game.)

One technique that sometimes helps is to take a nap in the morning and one in the afternoon; even ten or fifteen minutes will help. It also helps to give yourself plenty of time to sleep and, if your schedule allows it, to sleep until you wake up spontaneously in the morning.

If you have a serious case of narcolepsy, you should not drive or operate hazardous machinery until you are treated.

SUPPORT GROUPS

Besides a knowledgable and supportive physician, narcoleptics need support from others who share the same disease and therefore understand their problem. Information on narcolepsy and on support groups that have been formed in many cities is available from the American Narcolepsy Association, P.O. Box 1187, San Carlos, CA 94305 (1-800-222-6085; 1-800-222-6086 in California), and from the Narcolepsy Network, P.O. Box 1365, FDR Station, New York, NY 10150.

Periodic Movement of the Legs or Arms

People whose legs (or, occasionally, arms) jerk and twitch during sleep have a condition called *periodic limb movements*. Each twitch may last for 1 to 3 seconds, and the movements of the legs are spaced about 10 to 60 seconds apart. The episodes of twitching may last only a few minutes or they may continue for hours, with intervals of sound sleep in between; in severe cases, the twitches may occur throughout the night.

The movements themselves seem to do no damage, and some good sleepers have them without any problems. However if the twitches become strong or if they occur in a light sleeper, they can wake a person up. You don't realize what wakes you, because the twitch occurs before you awake.

If the periodic limb movements awaken you only a few times a night, you are likely to complain about insomnia. If the movements awaken you more frequently, you are more likely to complain about excessive daytime sleepiness. We know of one patient with severe excessive daytime sleepiness who found, to her surprise, that she had to replace her sheets about every three months because they were worn through by her feet. In the lab, she twitched at least 600 times each night, and each movement resulted in a few seconds of awakening of which she was totally unaware.

Up to a few years ago, periodic limb movements were called *nocturnal myoclonus*. However, myoclonus implies an epileptic mechanism, which this is not. We don't really know what causes the movements. There are likely to be many different causes. Occasionally, the twitches are caused by certain medications such as antidepressants (having your doctor make a switch in medicines might help) or by the withdrawal from other medication, such as tranquilizers and sedatives. Occasionally, poor circulation, a metabolic disease, kidney disease, or a folic acid deficiency may be implicated. But usually the cause is unknown.

Periodic limb movements increase with age. Researchers at the Veterans Administration Medical Center in San Diego found in studies of people aged 65 and older that one in three had this problem.

We are not talking here about the occasional whole-body jerk that occurs when you fall asleep. Nobody really understands what causes these sleep-onset jerks, but they are entirely without medical significance and not related to periodic limb movements.

TREATMENT

There is very little that can be done for periodic limb movements. There are some medications that suppress the twitches, and others that help you sleep through them—but they do not cure the twitches, and you may become habituated to the medications. Currently, the best medication seems to be Sinemet, a medication also prescribed for parkinsonism.

Some physicians have tried vitamin and mineral supplements, because they thought there might be some relationship, and they have had some success. There are no clinical studies on this, however. You might want to try supplements for a week or two and see if the twitches get better.

When poor peripheral circulation is suspected as a cause, you might try vitamin E supplements. Several clinical trials have shown that vitamin E increases peripheral circulation. Also, you could try a warm bath just before bedtime.

Restless-Legs Syndrome

Many people with periodic limb movements also have restless-legs syndrome (RLS), and almost all people with restless legs show periodic limb movements. With RLS, there are sensations deep within the leg muscles and knees that cause a powerful urge to move. One woman told her physician that she felt she must have bugs crawling in her muscles. When she moved, the bugs were still, but as soon as she sat down, she felt them start to crawl again. Luckily, the physician knew the syndrome and referred her to our sleep disorders center, where RLS was diagnosed.

Restless-legs syndrome alone usually causes difficulties falling asleep, rather than excessive daytime sleepiness. When combined with periodic leg movements, however, RLS often is associated with excessive daytime sleepiness.

Michael Malone, a 35-year-old electrician, had both restless legs and leg twitches. He said that he always felt washed out, and he had difficulties falling asleep because his legs were "nervous." He said he felt uncomfortable sensations creeping deep inside his legs when he relaxed. The urge to move his legs became so strong that he usually had to get up and walk for five or ten minutes before he could lie down again. Occasionally, the problem continued until 4 or 5 A.M. Even after sleeping an adequate number of hours, he felt unrefreshed. He often was unable to work, and he had to make do with jobs as a day laborer when he felt up to it.

Neurologic and psychiatric evaluations were negative. A sleep evaluation was performed on two consecutive nights. On each night, Mr. Malone got up twice after lights-outs to "walk off his legs." When he finally fell asleep about two hours after lights-out, episodes of periodic leg movements were recorded that awakened him about 350 times each night.

Mr. Malone was withdrawn from all stimulants, including coffee and tea. A gradually increasing exercise program was developed, including swimming and aerobics. He was placed on a number of different medications, each of which helped initially. When tolerance developed, he went off the medications for a few months at a time, alternating with months when he did take medication. That seemed to work.

In a number of cases, restless legs are associated with lack of exercise. Surprisingly, when exercise is started, the restless legs often become worse for a week or two before they get better. Occasionally, poor circulation seems to be involved; for example, in cases that are associated with pregnancy. Other cases have been traced to deficiencies, of iron, calcium, folic acid, or certain vitamins—especially vitamin E. Some cases have been related to various diseases, such as chronic uremia, diabetes, or metabolic diseases. In a remarkable number of cases, restless legs simply are a consequence of too much caffeine intake. About a third of RLS cases seem to have a hereditary factor.

TREATMENT

Self-help techniques include elimination of stimulants such as coffee, tea, and chocolate; a gradually increasing exercise program involving the legs; and exploration of iron, calcium, folic acid, and vitamin E supplements. If you do try supplements, we urge that you use a Sleep Log and try a week with and a week without each of the supplements, so that you can make an objective evaluation. Dr. M. I. Botez reports in the *Canadian Medical Association Journal* that several of his patients with RLS were shown to have a folate deficiency and recovered from their symptoms after taking folic acid supplements. Drs. Wayne Hening and Arthur Walters, of Lyons Veterans Administration Medical Center, report some success in treating RLS patients with opioids. Even on a long term basis, the opioids were taken at a low enough dosage that there was no addiction.

Consult your physician. There are some medications, such as Percodan and Tegretol, that can suppress the problem for a few weeks, although they do not cure it. Other drugs, such as Sinemet, are being investigated and may provide longer lasting relief.

Drug Side Effects

As discussed in Chapters 13 and 14, you can be excessively sleepy in the daytime as a side effect of some medication you are taking, such as antihistamines or tranquilizers. Excessive sleepiness also can be a side effect of a medication you have just *stopped* taking: For example, if you were taking a pill with a stimulant such as Dexedrine, various diet pills, heart medications, asthma medications, or birth control pills, and then you stop taking them, it may cause you to become very lethargic and sleepy for several days. Street drugs also can cause excessive daytime sleepiness.

TREATMENT

If you feel that any sleep problem (either excessive daytime sleepiness or insomnia) is associated with a medicine, ask your physician for advice in changing the dosage, trying an alternative medication, or gradually withdrawing from the medicine.

If ever a person is extremely sleepy or very difficult to arouse, it is important to get help immediately. If your physician cannot be reached, go to the emergency room of the nearest hospital or call a paramedic unit. Even if the reaction is to illegal drugs, it is better to go to the emergency room and face possible jail than it is to have somebody you know die.

Kleine-Levin Syndrome

The Kleine-Levin syndrome involves periodic excessive sleepiness that lasts for several weeks, alternating with apparently normal sleep. During the sleepy phases, a person may sleep as long as 20 to 22 hours per day. Strangely, at the same time, other drives are increased: The patient typically eats ferociously, drinks large amounts, and displays inappropriate sexual behavior. There also may be apathy, irritability, and confusion.

Kleine-Levin is a rare syndrome. It typically hits in the teens or early 20s and often disappears spontaneously during the 30s or 40s. More men than women suffer from it.

Many patients without Kleine-Levin have excessive sleepiness that waxes and wanes over periods of weeks or months. However, unless you also have an enormously increased appetite during those times when you are sleepy, it is unlikely that you have Kleine-Levin syndrome.

Menstrual-Related Hypersomnia

Since hormones such as estrogen and progesterone have a considerable influence on sleep, most women report sleeping better during some phases of their cycle than during others. Some patients have a monthly cycle of excessive daytime sleepiness that is so severe that they can barely remain awake for an eight-hour job. Others have insomnia during certain parts of their cycle.

In either of these cases, an endocrinologist or gynecologist, rather than a sleep specialist, should be consulted.

Parasomnias

Parasomnia refers to problems that occur during sleep, including such things as nightmares, bedwetting, and snoring.

Nightmares

Most people call anything a nightmare if it appears during sleep and is associated with anxiety. Sleep researchers, on the other hand, distinguish four different conditions: nightmares, sleep terrors, sleep-related panic attacks, and posttraumatic flashbacks.

Sleep researchers call a bad dream a nightmare if it arouses a person from REM sleep and if the person can remember the dream. Nightmares, while extremely frightening, usually do not result in much body reaction: The person does not sweat, the heart rate does not increase much, and breathing remains calm. Nightmares usually occur late in the night.

Edgar Allen Poe got many of his story plots from his nightmares.

Rose Wellington was a high-school senior planning to go to college, but was afraid that her repeated nightmares might expose her to ridicule in the dorm. Two or three times a week, she awakened early in the morning, fearful and agitated. She never screamed, but thrashed around in bed moaning and groaning, often awakening her sister. Her nightmares usually involved strangers lurking behind buildings, chasing her, grabbing her, and attempting to sexually assault her.

Psychological testing suggested that Rose was easily alarmed, somewhat immature, and starting to rebel against an overprotective family. Asked what she would do if attacked while awake, she thought about various options and finally decided that she would stab the man with a hat pin. We helped Rose rehearse this hat-pin scene repeatedly while she was awake. Rose also was enrolled in karate training to give her additional self-confidence. Within a few weeks, she had emerged victorious from a number of her nightmares; they soon disappeared, and she did fine in college.

Rose's story illustrates the essence of nightmares. They usually occur late at night, without much body involvement, and the person remembers a full dream. Nightmares suggest that some psychological problem or issue has not been resolved adequately (for example, what to do when attacked), and they often disappear when the problem is solved. Nightmares also can occur after withdrawal from medications, especially those that suppress REM sleep.

Sleep Terrors

Sleep terrors occur during delta sleep, the deepest sleep of the night. It is quite difficult to awaken from delta sleep. For some people, it is impossible. If such a person is disturbed in delta sleep, the brain becomes half asleep and half awake, and in that confused state, the sleep terror occurs.

Children have more delta sleep than do adults and therefore are more prone to sleep terrors. Because delta sleep is most abundant early at night, the sleep terror usually occurs within the first hour or so after falling asleep. It often starts with a bloodcurdling scream, and there is much body reaction—wide open eyes, rapidly beating heart, trembling, and sweating. The person is in obvious panic. It is difficult to talk to the person; he or she does not really know you are there. After a while, the victim curls up and falls asleep again—and almost always has forgotten the entire scene if asked about it the next morning. This is because the person never really awakens from sleep during a sleep terror.

Mark Trane was a 10-year-old who wanted to go to summer camp. However, his parents hesitated to send him because, three or four times a week, at about the parents' bedtime, Mark would wake up screaming, sweating, and wildly flailing his arms. He never remembered his sleep terrors in the morning. Mark's sleep terrors usually increased whenever he was under a new stress, and his parents were concerned that camp might increase their frequency.

Mark was observed in the sleep laboratory for two nights, mainly to rule out sleep-related epilepsy and other possible causes of his terrors. None were found. Psychological tests also were normal. The parents were advised to allow Mark plenty of sleep—because the more sleep there is, the less of it is delta (deep) sleep. For camp, 2 mg of Valium was prescribed to suppress delta sleep, to be taken just before going to bed. At this dosage, Mark had only one night terror during the four-week camp. When the Valium was withdrawn after camp, the night terrors briefly reappeared, but then became infrequent. They reappeared dramatically when he was transferred to a new school, then disappeared again when he became more comfortable there.

You can easily distinguish nightmares from sleep terrors: Sleep terrors occur early at night, nightmares much later; sleep terrors show much bodily agitation, nightmares do not; people remember only short fragments from a sleep terror, but remember long and frightening dreams from the nightmares.

In children, it is important to make the distinction, because a child who has frequent nightmares might need psychotherapy, but a child with sleep terrors usually does not. Sleep terrors in adults are more serious. They often indicate excessive agitation, anxiety, and sometimes aggressive impulses. Therefore, adults who have frequent sleep terrors might do well to talk to a psychiatrist.

Sleep terrors in children can make it difficult for a child to go to camp or on an overnight. In that case, it can be helpful to abolish the sleep terrors temporarily with low doses of Valium. We do not advise Valium for chronic use, but you might test it for a night or two at home before sending the child off to his or her social event, to see whether the dosage is adequate and to give the child confidence.

Occasionally, sleep terrors are caused by certain medications or the withdrawal from certain medications. If this a possibility, discuss it with your physician.

Persons who have sleep terrors should try to decrease their delta sleep by sleeping longer hours. (The longer you sleep, the more shallow your sleep becomes—something to be avoided by people who have insomnia, but encouraged in people who have sleep terrors.)

Sleep-Related Panic Attacks

· · ● ● ● · ·

In some research I did with Drs. Matthew Friedman and Charles Ra-
varis at Dartmouth Medical School, we studied patients who suffer from
daytime panic attacks. In such patients, extreme episodes of panic—in-
cluding breathing difficulties, racing heart, sweating, trembling, and
fear of dying or going insane—occur during wakefulness. Sometimes, the
attacks seem to be triggered by certain events such as being in a crowd;
other times, there doesn't seem to be a triggering event. Such patients
also may suffer from nighttime panic attacks that awaken them from
sleep. Typically, these nighttime panic attacks do not occur during REM
sleep, as do the nightmares, nor during delta sleep, as do the sleep ter-
rors, but during stage 2 or 3 sleep.

· · ● ● ● · ·

Posttraumatic Stress Disorder

Patients who suffer from posttraumatic stress disorder occasionally
have flashbacks and anxiety attacks at the transition point between
waking and sleeping (in stage 1 or light stage 2). So this is an entirely
different type of "nightmare."

In panic attacks and flashbacks, psychiatric treatment of the daytime problem is considered more effective than focusing on the nighttime events.

Night Sweats

Persistent night sweats are a red flag for physicians, because they may
be a sign of several serious diseases, such as tuberculosis, thyroid
infection, and malaria. Night sweats also are frequent during menopause. If you wake up with night sweats, lower your room temperature
or sleep with fewer covers. Check your temperature to see whether
you are running a fever. If not, and if the night sweats are frequent,
see your doctor for a workup.

Sleep Talking

People may talk in their sleep either during REM (dreaming) sleep or during an incomplete arousal from delta (deep) sleep. If you talk during REM sleep, your pronunciation is clear and understandable. Delta sleep talking is much more mumbled and unintelligible.

Usually during REM sleep, all muscles except those of the eyes are paralyzed. Occasionally, however, the speech muscles escape this paralysis, and simply talk out the things we are dreaming about.

Sometimes a sleep talker also can hear what someone in the awake world says, often incorporating it into the dream and answering. Sleep talkers almost never remember talking in their sleep, even if you wake them up immediately after the episode.

Sleep Paralysis

Muscle paralysis during the daytime is known as *cataplexy;* similar muscle paralysis when falling asleep or upon awakening is known as *sleep paralysis.* The victim cannot move any muscles except those of the eyes and sometimes feels like snakes or bugs are crawling over the body. The paralysis may last about two to five minutes.

Sleep-onset paralysis often is a symptom of narcolepsy. Paralysis upon awakening, although frightening, is benign and does not indicate any disease.

If you experience sleep paralysis, you can speed up the return of muscle tone by blinking your eyes rapidly, rotating them in circles, and moving them from side to side and up and down. Then, contract the muscles in your face and around your mouth, moving your jaw and your tongue; as tone returns, start moving your neck, shoulders, arms, fingers, legs, ankles, and toes. Sit up and move all the muscles again.

Leg Cramps

Leg cramps at night can be a rude awakening, with severe pain in the sole of the foot or in the muscles of the calf. The cramps often occur in women when they switch from wearing low-heeled shoes to high heels, and vice versa.

For immediate relief, some people find massage helpful. Others need to get up, walk around, and shake their legs to get the muscles to relax. It may help to do a calf-stretching exercise: Stand facing a wall two or three feet away, place your hands on the wall, and lean forward, keeping your heels on the floor and your legs straight. You will feel a pulling sensation in the calf muscles. Hold the position for ten seconds. Relax for five seconds and repeat. If cramps occur frequently, do the exercise three times a day until you no longer have the nighttime cramps.

Leg cramps also may be caused by a potassium deficiency, especially from taking diuretic medications, or by calcium or magnesium deficiencies. If you have leg cramps frequently, you may want to take potassium, calcium, and magnesium supplements to see if this makes a difference. One Florida doctor reports that raising the head of his bed about nine inches on wood blocks eliminated his leg cramps.

Sleepwalking (Somnambulism)

Sleepwalking is quite common: According to the American Medical Association, some 4 million Americans have sought medical help for sleepwalking.

It was once believed that sleepwalkers were acting out dreams, but this has been proven untrue. Rather, sleepwalking is caused by the same mechanism that causes sleep terrors: incomplete arousal from delta sleep.

During a sleepwalking episode, the brain is half awake and half asleep. Occasionally, it can carry out simple operations such as avoiding obstacles, but it also can be confused, so the sleepwalker falls down the stairs or mistakes a window for a door.

There are stories of sleepwalkers driving cars, boarding planes, going swimming, and performing other complex actions. This is unlikely. Although sleepwalkers, in their confused state, might be able to enter a car and start it, they would not have the fast reflexes needed to drive and probably would crash the car before getting out of the driveway.

To decrease the risk of self-harm, sleepwalkers should, if possible, sleep on the first floor. Also, when there is a sleepwalker in the house, put away dangerous objects and car keys and consider installing a special latch on the door.

Sleepwalking is quite common in children, but they usually outgrow the condition as they get older. As with sleep terrors, sleepwalking happens more often during periods of tension and anxiety, but children who sleepwalk are psychologically as healthy as children who do not. There seems to be some inherited component: Children are much more likely to sleepwalk if their parents did.

Sleepwalking in adults is more worrisome. Extreme stress, anxiety, and—occasionally—epilepsy are possible causes. Therefore, adults with this problem should seek medical help, possibly coupled with relaxation training and biofeedback. Occasionally, hypnosis works.

Some medications may help. Valium, Tofranil, and some stimulants have abolished sleepwalking in some cases. In cases where nighttime epilepsy is found to be the cause, anticonvulsants are useful.

Bedwetting (Enuresis)

Bedwetting is relatively common in children. At age 5, about 10 percent of girls and 15 percent of boys still wet the bed frequently. This means only that they are somewhat slow in maturing—if nothing is done, they usually gain control as they become older. Occasionally, some people continue to wet their beds in adulthood. One study showed a 1 to 3 percent rate of bedwetting in apparently healthy Navy recruits.

Sometimes a child has been dry for a few months and then starts to wet the bed again. This usually is a clue that the bedwetting is due to some psychological disturbance, such as the arrival of a new baby brother or sister. Bedwetting also can be caused by a urinary tract or kidney disorder or a hormonal upset. It can be a symptom of an infection, pinworms, diabetes, epilepsy, or sickle cell anemia.

TREATMENT

Never punish or shame a child for bed wetting. If the child is old enough, let him or her take care of the problem as much as possible. Being able to change the bed and wash the sheets helps rebuild the badly wounded feeling of self-esteem.

Avoid an excessive intake of fluid in the late afternoon and early evening. See that the child always empties the bladder before going to bed. If you wake the child to urinate before you go to bed, make sure that the child is fully awake. Letting the child sleep while you guide him or her to the bathroom only teaches that one can urinate while sleeping. Have a rug at the foot of the bed to make it easier to leave the warm bed and a night-light or two to show the way.

Dr. Nathan Azrin, professor of psychology at Nova University in Fort Lauderdale, and his colleagues have developed an effective one-day program for bedwetters. On the chosen day, practice sessions are held every half hour to rehearse what the child should do at night: The child lies down in bed and, at the word *go*, jumps up and goes to the bathroom. That night, the parent awakens the child every hour for the first few hours to go to the bathroom. In 55 children who were bedwetters, this method dramatically decreased bedwetting, the average child having four accidents in two weeks after training and then being dry. Only one in five later started wetting again, and most of these improved with a second practice session.

Another approach is bladder stretching. When the child is at home during the day, encourage him or her to drink large amounts of fluids. Then ask the child to hold his or her urine for as long as possible. Do this every day and give rewards for longer periods of bladder control. This technique helps the child to gain control of the bladder muscles.

Stream-interruption exercises (voluntarily starting and stopping urine flow) also can increase control by increasing tone of the sphincter muscles.

The bell-and-pad method works in many cases. When urine is released, a bell sounds, awakening the sleeper. After a few nights, the sleeper hopefully learns to awaken before the bell rings. Summarizing the results of 40 studies involving more than 1,000 children shows a success rate of about 75 percent.

Whatever method is used, be sure to include emotional support and rewards. Try to diminish stress and excitement in the household. Talk the problem over with your child. Don't rush him or her. Don't scold, nag, threaten, or suggest that the behavior is shameful or dirty. Self-assurance and love are more effective. Most important is to relax and help the child get a sense of honor and faith in himself or herself in other areas.

If a child who wets the bed is going to camp or visiting overnight, medication such as imipramine may be helpful. However, bedwetting usually returns when the drug is stopped. Talk to the child's pediatrician.

Especially in adult bedwetters, try eliminating caffeine from the diet. As we said earlier, more than 60 percent of cases of incontinence due to caffeine have been reported, and the urgency to urinate often can be overcome simply by eliminating caffeine from the diet.

One cause of bedwetting and frequent urination in men is an enlarged prostate. (The prostate is a horseshoe-shaped gland about the size of a walnut that encircles the lower neck of the bladder. When enlarged, it can press against the bladder.) Prostate enlargement can be treated by surgery and also can be helped by quitting smoking, eliminating caffeine, reducing alcohol and fat from the diet, increasing exercise, and reducing weight if you are overweight.

If a child or an adult experiences pain when urinating, has blood in the urine, urinates very frequently, or dribbles urine in the daytime, consult a physician right away.

Sleep-Related Bruxism (Tooth-Grinding)

Some people grind their teeth only at night; others do it both during the day and at night, often when they're under particular stress.

Patients usually have no awareness of grinding their teeth at night; however, it can cause awakenings and a complaint of insomnia, an aching jaw, or headaches. Often a dentist can spot the problem, because the tooth surfaces usually show excessive wear.

If you grind your teeth during the day, biofeedback often can help, but it is less useful in nighttime grinding. Where grinding is related to malocclusion of the teeth, the problem can be corrected orthodontically. If nothing else can be done, patients can wear rubber mouth guards to prevent tooth damage.

Sleep-Related Epilepsy

In one out of four people who have epilepsy, their seizures occur mainly at night. These nighttime seizures, called *sleep epilepsy*, can occur at all ages, but are most common in children. They can be the cause of bedwetting, sleepwalking, or other body movements (these things, of course, also can occur in the absence of epilepsy). If you suspect epilepsy, a neurologist should be consulted.

A standard study in a sleep lab does not diagnose sleep-related epilepsy because, typically, not enough EEG electrodes are used and the paper is run at too slow a speed. However, if a sleep-related seizure disorder is suspected, a full clinical EEG can be run at night to evaluate the problem.

Sleep-Related Gastroesophageal Reflux

Although there is a sphincter to prevent it, gastric juices sometimes enter the esophagus from the stomach. This is called *gastroesophageal reflux* and often is felt as heartburn. It sometimes happens after a heavy meal or, less commonly, during sleep. Patients also may have a hiatal hernia, in which part of the stomach is above the sphincter and acid sometimes spills up into the esophagus, causing serious heartburn.

TREATMENT

Sleep with the head of the bed elevated. (Put six-inch wooden blocks underneath the legs at the head of the bed.)

Reduce stress in your life.

Avoid high-fat meals and highly acid or spicy foods.

Lose weight if you are overweight, and do not wear garments that constrict the waist or abdomen.

If these measures do not help, medications can be given, either antacids or medications to help with faster clearing of the acid (such as Bethanechol) or to suppress acid secretion by the stomach during the night.

Sleep-Related Headaches

There are three types of headache frequently associated with sleep: migraine headache, cluster headache, and chronic paroxysmal hemicrania. Migraine headaches usually occur only on one side of the head and may be accompanied by nausea, vomiting, and sensory disturbances. In cluster headaches, the pain typically focuses around one eye. The name *cluster* derives from the fact that the headaches come in clusters—headache-free periods alternate with periods of excruciatingly painful headache. Chronic paroxysmal hemicrania involves short-lasting headaches, but they occur more frequently than do cluster headaches.

Although there is still debate, it appears that when these headaches occur when you wake from sleep, often in the early morning hours, they are related to REM sleep. During NREM sleep, especially delta sleep, blood vessels to the brain are constricted. During REM sleep, these blood vessels dilate, causing a greatly increased flow of blood to the brain. This dilation causes the headache. The pain comes from stretch receptors located within the walls of the blood vessels. The more constricted the blood vessels become during NREM sleep, the more they dilate during REM sleep.

TREATMENT

Most people who suffer from sleep-related headaches need to be treated with medication. However, reducing stress also can be helpful. The less tense you get during the day, the less your blood vessels constrict and the less they need to dilate later. Also, don't deprive yourself of sleep—for example, by working or partying very late— because cutting down on time in bed increases delta sleep, the most intense NREM sleep. Since a less intense NREM sleep means less vasoconstriction and therefore a less intense rebound dilation during REM sleep, it makes sense to let yourself sleep long and regularly. Naps may help.

SUNDAY MORNING HEADACHE

Headache on Sunday morning might be caused by excessive week-end partying with alcohol, but it also can be caused by caffeine with-drawal. If you usually drink several cups of coffee in the morning, sleeping late means you are getting less caffeine.

Try cutting back on your coffee intake during the week.

Sleep-related morning headaches also may be associated with sleep apnea.

Sleep-Related Laryngospasm

Occasionally, patients wake up with an inability to breathe, a feeling of choking, and stridor (high-pitched noise made during breathing). Typically, the episodes stop after about a minute or so, but they are associated with anxiety and agitation. These episodes are caused by spasms in your larynx—you can't get air in or out of your lungs. The condition is not related to sleep aphea.

Sleep-related laryngospasm needs to be differentiated from night-time panic attacks and from sleep terrors. In sleep-related laryngospasm, the difficulty is related only to breathing; or in some cases, the spasms may be related to gastroesophageal reflux. Try the measures suggested for that condition.

REM Behavior Disorder

Ordinarily, all our muscles are paralyzed just before we start dreaming. The brain does not know that we are dreaming and gives our muscles the commands to move, but our bodies do not do it. For example, when we dream of running, our leg muscles are commanded to run; luckily, because they are paralyzed, they can manage only very small twitches.

Occasionally, for unknown reasons, the muscle paralysis is not total, and people then carry out part of their dreams. They might bolt straight up in bed, fling themselves around, or hit the pillow. Occasionally, they hurt themselves or others with these activities.

There are some medications that seem to help. However, it also is important that patients with REM behavior disorder do everything possible to prevent hurting themselves or others. They might put their mattress on the floor, have the floor thickly carpeted, place furniture and lamps far away, and consider sleeping alone.

Rhythmic Movement Disorder

Some people rock in their sleep, or they bang their head rhythmically. We know of an 8-year-old who rocks so violently when trying to fall asleep that he moves his bed clear across the room. Similarly, a 46-year-old executive we know has the habit, awake or asleep, of sitting up in bed three or four times each night and gently swaying his body back and forth for about ten minutes. If he is left alone, he sleeps soundly the rest of the night. If his habit is interfered with, he has difficulties sleeping.

Rhythmic movements typically increase with stress. In a case recorded for three nights in our laboratory, a 12-year-old boy rocked for about 2-1/2 hours on the first night, for about 45 minutes on the second, and for only 10 minutes on the third. This rocking occurred when he was awake and also during the lighter stages of sleep.

It is possible that some cases of rhythmic movement disorder have a neurologic basis. However, in most patients, they seem to be simply comfort habits, much like thumbsucking as with thumbsucking, there is debate about whether rhythmic movements should be aggressively stopped to break the habit or left undisturbed. In many cases, the rhythmic movements can be stopped if they are prevented from occurring for a number of weeks, such as by having a parent hold the child quietly so that he or she cannot rock. However, those weeks are unhappy and tense, and most children outgrow the behavior even without treatment.

Snoring

"Laugh and the world laughs with you, snore and you sleep alone," said Anthony Burgess.

People who snore have at least one of the following problems:

1. Low muscle tone in the muscles of the tongue and throat. (Alcohol and other drugs relax these muscles even further, causing increased snoring.)
2. Excessive bulkiness of tissue in the throat, such as large tonsils and adenoids, big uvulas, or excessive length of the soft palate.
3. Obstructed nasal airways. When the mucous membranes become stuffy and swollen, the air passage becomes smaller. You then have to breathe with exaggerated force to move the air through the narrow hole. This explains why some people snore only during hayfever season or when they have a cold.
4. Anatomical deformities in the airway. Some people have a broken or crooked nose, which cuts down on the airway size. Being overweight also can cause snoring, because fat deposits around the upper airway make the airway smaller.

About half of all adults snore occasionally, and one out of four snores regularly. Snoring is much more prevalent in men than in women until menopause, when almost as many women as men start snoring. Children seldom snore unless they have enlarged tonsils or adenoids.

Habitual snorers are twice as likely to have high blood pressure as are nonsnorers. And, of course, snoring often is associated with sleep apnea.

TREATMENT

Try increasing the humidity in your bedroom. Dry and swollen membranes can cause snoring.

Check for allergies. They can cause swelling of tissue. One patient stopped snoring after he eliminated wheat from his diet, because he was allergic to it.

Try to sleep on your side. Most people snore more when sleeping on their backs.

Avoid smoking and drinking, both of which can bring on snoring.

Be sure to exercise regularly. It will help you lose excess weight.

Avoid tranquilizers and sleeping pills before bedtime.

There are more than 300 antisnoring devices registered at the U.S. Patent Office. There are chin and head straps, neck collars, jaw braces to keep the jaw from falling back, and electrical devices to produce unpleasant stimuli when the patient snores. They seem to work in some cases, but not many. Some are dangerous, possibly causing injury. Talk to your doctor before buying any expensive device.

Surgery to increase airflow in the airway—such as removing tonsils, or correcting a deviated septum, or eliminating extra tissue—can help with snoring. The UPPP (uvulopalatopharyngoplasty), discussed in relation to sleep apnea, can be quite helpful to people with a severe snoring problem.

Nonrestorative Sleep

Nonrestorative sleep is classified neither as a disorder of excessive daytime sleepiness nor as a parasomnia. People who have nonrestorative sleep wake up in the morning after apparently good sleep and are still tired and not refreshed. They are more sensitive to pain in the morning than they were in the evening, and they have malaise—that is, they just generally don't feel good even though they do not have any specific places where they clearly hurt. They often feel stiff, like patients with rheumatoid arthritis. Indeed, if such patients go to an internist, they will probably be diagnosed as having *fibrositis* (also known as *fibromyalgia*), a term used to denote arthritislike symptoms without other physical signs of the arthritis. If the same people talk to a psychiatrist, they might be classified as having hypochondria, because they have vague complaints without there being objective evidence for any disease.

• • ● ● • •

In a study that I did with Dr. David Hawkins at the University of Virginia in Charlottesville in 1973, we noticed that some insomniac patients did not show the expected EEG waves during NREM sleep, the sleep during which body recovery should occur best. Rather, such people showed a mixture of delta NREM sleep waves and alpha waves, the waves that denote relaxed wakefulness. In other words, throughout the night, according to the brain waves, they were somehow both asleep and awake at the same time. We coined the term alpha-delta sleep *for this type of sleep. We observed that the patients who showed this kind of sleep often suffered from the chronic malaise we have been talking about.*

Dr. Harvey Moldofsky from the Clark Institute in Toronto then studied a group of patients with fibrositis and found that they all showed this intrusion of alpha (waking) waves into NREM sleep. He called it nonrestorative sleep, *speculating that such patients do sleep, but get very little benefit from it.*

In another study, Dr. Moldofsky disturbed the sleep of healthy volunteers by sounding tones frequently when they were in NREM sleep. Because of these tones, the volunteers could sleep uninterrupted for only short periods. After each tone, their sleeping waves were mixed with alpha (waking) waves. In the morning, the volunteers complained about the same type of malaise as did the patients with fibrositis. Dr. Modolfsky thought that it was the mixing of alpha (waking) and NREM sleep waves that caused such patients to have the morning symptoms.

Dr. Moldofsky then found that athletes did not show the expected morning stiffness and malaise when their sleep was disturbed all night. This led to the conclusion that if you are fit and exercise regularly, you can overcome some of the symptoms of nonrestorative sleep.

In another study, it was shown that very low dosages of the antidepressant Elavil (10 to 25 mg) often clear away the alpha intrusions from the sleep EEG—apparently not because such patients are depressed, but because Elavil subtly changes brain chemistry and this somehow helps the "sleep-wake switch" to be thrown more firmly toward sleep, rather than being stuck in the middle. Other antidepressants might work, too, but have not yet been tried in the research labs.

In yet another study, it was found that nonrestorative sleep often starts during a period of stress. When stressed, we have many more awakenings and, therefore, the chance of mixing alpha and sleeping waves becomes greater. In many cases, this mixing persists, even after the stress has disappeared.

· · ● ● ● · · ·

Cause-effect relationships are not clear. People with pain wake up more during the night and produce more of this alpha-delta mixture in their brain waves. Vice versa, when the alpha-delta mixture is artificially produced by awakening healthy sleepers, it aggravates any pain that the patient might have. So it seems to be a vicious circle, sleep and pain each aggravating the other.

When nonrestorative sleep is a problem, three things usually are prescribed. The first is a low dose of Elavil, the second is exercise and the third is counseling. Because patients usually feel as if they have arthritis, a very gentle, gradually increasing amount of exercise should be planned. We do not recommend jogging or other jarring exercise, but we do recommend swimming, low-impact aerobics, or walking. Finally, because the disorder often starts with a period of stress, some supportive therapy or a sympathetic, understanding physician often is an important part of the treatment.

···· 16 ····

When You Need Further Help

We hope that you have followed the steps in this program and are now among the more than 80 percent of the people who are helped by the guidelines we have outlined. A few people, however, probably will need further help. How can you tell whether you are among them?

You should seek further help if:

- Your insomnia has continued for six months or more, is seriously affecting your daytime functioning, and this program has not helped after you have given it a good try
- Your sleep problem has caused an accident or near-accident at work, at home, or on the road
- Your sleep problem has jeopardized a job or a social relationship
- You feel or someone else says that there is something abnormal about your sleep—such as breathing difficulties, leg twitching, or bed-wetting
- You have great difficulty staying awake during the day
- You experience marked mental difficulties—such as forgetfulness or disorientation—along with your sleep problem

If any of these problems exist, you should talk to your doctor. If your doctor can't help, you need a referral to a sleep disorders center. In any case, if your problem is serious and chronic and you can't handle it—whether it's that you can't get to sleep, can't stay asleep, or can't stay awake during the day—get help.

Chronic is the key word here. You don't need professional help for short term problems—most people occasionally sleep poorly for a week or a month. But if your problem continues and you have tried everything you can on this program, don't suffer needlessly—get help.

The longer you go on thinking that nothing can be done about your insomnia, the more difficult it will be to treat it.

Where to Go

Remember that poor sleep can have medical causes. If nothing you have tried seems to work and you have not yet seen a physician, you should see one to evaluate your medical health. Be sure to tell the physician the total history of your problem and everything that you have done to try to solve it. Don't accept a quick prescription for a sleeping pill, but ask for a thorough evaluation for possible causes.

If you feel that stress, anxiety, or a recent emotional shock are the basis of your poor sleep, and you have not been able to solve the problem on your own, you may want to consult with a stress-management consultant or a psychiatrist, psychologist, or other mental-health professional.

Your family doctor can recommend an appropriate therapist, or you can go to a mental health center or walk-in clinic. Talk to them about the services and approaches they offer and then decide whether you think one of those approaches is right for you. You also could contact the psychiatry department of a nearby medical school or hospital. Or you can get a personal recommendation from somebody who has benefited from working with a particular psychiatrist or clinical psychologist in private practice. Most schools and colleges have psychological services for students that are free or low cost. If you drink much alcohol or use drugs, you can go to a facility specializing in drug and alcohol treatment.

You may want to choose a psychiatrist (an M.D. who is a specialist in the treatment of mental illnesses), especially if you think there could be a biological as well as a psychological aspect to your problem. As a physician, a psychiatrist can prescribe drugs. If you feel that you basically need counseling, you could choose a psychologist (a Ph.D. who often is specifically trained in behavior therapy, but cannot prescribe drugs). And there are other sources of help: your clergyman, a marriage counselor, a social worker in a hospital or at a social agency, a biofeedback specialist, or a stress-management consultant.

You may want to choose individual help, or enter group therapy to discuss your problems with other people under the supervision of a professional. You also could join a group such as Alcoholics Anonymous, Addicts Anonymous, Gamblers Anonymous, Neurotics Anonymous, or Recovery. If it is an emergency, you can even use a telephone counseling service that has a hot line for medical or psychiatric help. There are special numbers for alcoholics or drug addicts, for persons who are thinking about suicide, and for general counseling with any emotional problem. Check your local telephone book.

When You Should Go to a Sleep Disorders Center

For some conditions, a sleep specialist should be your first stop after you talk to your doctor. Unexplained excessive daytime sleepiness and nonrestorative sleep are two such conditions. If your bed partner suggests that you might have symptoms of sleep apnea, other breathing difficulty, or frequent leg twitches or other movements during sleep, you should go to a sleep disorders center. Finally, you should go to a center, if as an insomniac, you have investigated possible psychological problems, poor sleep hygiene, lifestyle problems, and medical conditions, and still have not been helped.

If You Go to a Sleep Disorders Center

Once you've decided to go to a center, how do you get in? It's usually best to get a referral from your physician. That way, the center won't need to repeat tests that have already been done by your doctor and can refer its findings back to him or her. However, some centers will make appointments directly with patients.

The appendix of this book contains the official list of centers accredited by the American Sleep Disorders Association (ASDA). This means that they have been checked by the ASDA and are accepted as being knowledgeable in the field and meeting ASDA's high standards. There are also sources to contact for lists of centers in other countries.

Most sleep disorders centers look pretty much alike and do about the same things. Usually, you'll be sent a Sleep Log and a Sleep Questionnaire. Once you have filled out the questionnaire and kept the log for a week or two, and your doctor has sent the center a summary of your medical record, the center will set up an interview. (We suggest that you also send or take the Sleep Logs, Day Logs, and answers to the questionnaires in this book.)

At the interview, a sleep specialist will ask you questions to find out more about how you sleep, psychological and social issues, and your ideas and feelings about your sleep problem. It's important to be forthright with the sleep specialist. Small details can be important and, no matter how unusual or personal you think something is, your counselor probably has heard it before. If you leave something out, that one fact could be the key to evaluating your problem.

After the interview, which may last half an hour to two hours, the specialist will decide if you need to sleep overnight in the lab. Most insomniacs don't need to sleep in the lab; you'll only have to do this if an evaluation needs to be made of periodic limb movements or other physical factors.

If you do sleep in the lab, you might be asked to stay the following day to complete a multiple sleep latency test (MSLT). This test will measure how sleepy you are during the day. You'll go to bed at two-hour intervals for about 20 minutes, and the center will measure whether and how fast you fall asleep.

Finally, you may have a follow-up visit with the sleep specialist to discuss the center's findings and recommendations for your insomnia. Or, if you were referred by a physician, the center might simply report this information to your physician.

If You Sleep in the Lab

Many people ask, "How can I ever sleep in the lab with wires attached to me and somebody watching me, when I can't even sleep at home?"

In our experience, this is almost never a problem. In fact, many insomniacs sleep much better in the lab than at home, and it's hard to find what's wrong with their sleep when they sleep so well. There are many reasons for this. Some people simply give up and plan just to lie there and not even try to sleep. Of course, as we discussed before, the less you try to sleep, the more easily you can. Other people are so relieved that someone is taking an active interest in their insomnia that they sleep better. Some patients are conditioned against sleeping in their own bedrooms and so sleep better in the lab. Some people feel safer and more secure in the lab, and others sleep better away from the noises and the aggravations at home.

Even if you turn out to be the rare person who dose have trouble sleeping in the lab, it's okay—you're there so they can find out about your bad sleep. You'll be giving them plenty to measure and study.

If You Come

You should not take any naps during the day before coming to the lab. Unless otherwise instructed, do not use alcohol, stimulants, or sedatives 24 hours before the study, and don't drink any coffee or tea after breakfast. Check with the sleep disorders center on what to do about other medications you take regularly. You may eat a normal evening meal before coming. Bring comfortable sleep attire (with robe and socks or slippers for walking around the halls or sitting in the TV room if there is one) and personal hygiene items you need at bedtime and in the morning. When you get to your room, you will be asked to fill out a presleep questionnaire that asks what you have done during the day and whether you took any medication that day or recently.

What They Do

After you get into your pajamas and are ready for bed, a sleep technician will attach various electrodes. These are little metal cups smaller than a dime, filled with jelly and attached to very flexible wires. The first ones are attached to your head and measure the brain waves that you are creating both while you are awake and through your various sleep stages. Depending on the lab, there may be anywhere from two to six electrodes that are glued onto your scalp with collodion or some other substance. (The collodion can be removed the next morning with acetone; if any is still left, you can use nail-polish remover at home to get it out.)

There also may be attachments to each of your earlobes as neutral controls. The earlobe is almost the only place on the head where not much is going on; there is no muscle tension, eye movement, brain waves, or anything else, so the earlobe is used for a neutral reference.

An ear oxymeter may be attached to the earlobe to measure how well your blood is saturated with oxygen. As you may know, when blood carries more oxygen it is redder, and when blood carries less oxygen, it is bluer. With the ear oxymeter, a light is shone into your earlobe and the oxymeter measures the color of the reflected light.

From that, we can determine how well your blood is oxygenated during sleep. If you have apnea, this often helps to determine how serious the apnea might be.

There will be other electrodes alongside your eyes to measure your eye movements (electro-oculogram or EOG). Electrodes on your chin will measure muscle tension and relaxation (electromyogram or EMG). The EMG is especially important during REM sleep to see whether your muscles are paralyzed, as they should be in REM sleep.

Sensors are placed in front of your nostrils to measure the temperature and airflow just outside your nose. (The temperature is cooler when you inhale and warmer when you exhale, and from this we can tell whether you are actually moving air or not.) Two bands usually are applied to measure breathing movement, one around your abdomen and one around your chest. With these bands, we can get a feeling for how much air is actually being moved, or whether you are trying to breathe, but cannot, because you have sleep apnea caused by some obstruction. (Some labs measure the same thing with electrodes that are applied to the skin between the ribs, where they measure muscle contractions and relaxations when you try to breathe.)

Electrodes are applied to your legs to measure whether or not your legs are twitching during sleep. Finally, electrodes will be placed on your chest or back to record your electrocardigram (EKG).

All these measurements are more or less standard for any patient in any lab. But sometimes there are additions and variations. For example, if there is a chance that you might be having seizures at night, you will have extra electrodes applied to your scalp to make additional measurements of brain waves. If you are suspected of having sleep apnea, and we cannot get a reasonable recording of your breathing from the bands around the chest and the abdomen (perhaps because you are too heavy), a small balloon on a plastic tube might be inserted through your nose and fairly far down into your throat to measure the pressure there and assess breathing effort. That is done very rarely, however, and it is much less painful than it sounds.

You will sleep in a regular bed in a private bedroom, and there will be a closet to hang your clothes. Your wires will be plugged into special outlets at the head of your bed, feeding into various recording instruments in the monitoring room. This room looks like a mini-version of Mission Control, with recording instruments busily tracing the physiology of each patient as he or she sleeps. Technicians monitor the recordings from this room. They keep an all-night vigil, charting the brain activity as each sleeper passes through the various stages of sleep. Then, they calculate various measurements for the sleep specialists to study the next morning.

(You might want to know that in an accredited sleep lab, the technicians who work with you are well trained. There is now an association—the Association of Polysomnographic Technologists—that gives exams, and many of the technicians who work with you have been certified by that organization. They know what they are doing, and you are in safe hands in the lab. Probably you are safer there than if you were sleeping at home, because somebody is always awake in the lab making sure everything is okay.)

Don't worry that you might receive a shock from any of the wires attached to you. The instruments are set up to measure the electricity that *you* produce—they don't put out any electricity that could shock you.

Once the EEG electrodes are connected, the technician flips a switch, and at least eight pens start scratching back and forth on a moving stack of paper, making long, scribbly lines of waves and peaks and wiggles. You and the technician talk back and forth on the microphone in your room for a few minutes to test the quality of the recordings. The technician makes checks with your eyes open and closed, while moving your eyes to the right and left, while breathing, while holding your breath, while tensing and relaxing your leg muscles, and so on.

In your bed, you can move around easily and twist and turn as much as you want—the electrodes are attached to very flexible wires. You do have to get unplugged to go the bathroom, because the wires are not that long. But don't worry, in all sleep disorders centers there is a technician on duty all night monitoring the equipment, and your room microphone will be turned on all night near you. If you want to get up, you simply call, and the technician comes and unplugs the wires so you can go to the bathroom. Don't worry about how often you need to call for assistance. Some patients are so nervous that they have to go the bathroom 10 or 15 times, and it's the technician's job to unplug you however many times you need to get up.

Some laboratories have setups for video recording, so there might be a dim light or an infrared light and a video camera in your room. That is because the technicians need to know what positions you lie in during the night. Some people snore only on their backs, and some people twitch violently while sleeping. Some labs also have specially designed position monitors that measure in what position you are lying.

The Record

The recordings are inked across a long, continuous paper about two feet wide and about a thousand feet long. Near the bottom are the regular waves of your breathing, and in the middle are the typical spikes of the EKG. Further up usually come recordings of sounds and body movements, and on the top is the recording of the EEG and the eye movements. These recordings are called a *polysomnogram,* which is much more complicated and measures many more aspects of your body than does an EKG.

As the pen traces out the brain waves of the EEG, the waves first are fast and small, indicating that you are awake. When you get drowsy, regular and larger waves appear, about ten per second. In the transition between sleeping and waking, the waves become slower, about three to seven per second. The first signs on the EEG that you are actually asleep are the sleep spindles, displaying quick bursts of rapid waves, like crescendos and decrescendos in a musical performance. As you fall asleep, the recordings of the eye movements show slow rolls as the eyes move back and forth. You can see typical recordings in the figure on page 14.

Soon, the record shows bursts of spindle waves interspersed with larger slow waves, occurring at about one per second. These large waves, called delta waves, become more frequent, the sleeper rarely moves, and the person is in deep delta sleep. This is the best sleep of the night, when most bodily recovery occurs. Depending on your age, your physical fitness, and how long you have been awake before going to bed, you might spend 5 to 90 minutes in this delta sleep.

Then you retrace the sequence. The delta waves drop out, and about 90 minutes after you fell asleep, you enter a new stage. Your brain waves begin to look as if you are almost awake. Your eyes move under your closed lids, as if you're looking around. You are dreaming, and your muscles are paralyzed to prevent you from carrying out your dreams. This is REM sleep.

As the night goes on, you have less and less delta sleep, and a dream occurs about every 90 minutes. The first one lasts only about 5 minutes and usually is boring, a rehash of something you did that day. Every dream gets a little longer and more exciting than the previous one. If you sleep six hours a night, you probably have four dreams.

Another thing we see on the EEG is that everybody, even the best sleeper, wakes up 10 to 15 times each night. The difference is that the good sleepers fall back to sleep within a few seconds and later do not even remember that they have been awake. The poor sleepers, on the other hand, stay awake much longer and remember it.

Things are not quiet in the land of Morpheus. The average sleeper—quiet, passive—hardly betrays the busy brain activity going on within. But in the sleep labs, EEG recordings clearly document this activity. As one sleep researcher said, "It's not like parking your brain in the garage for the night. Things are going on!"

The EEG brain-wave charts represent the brain's computing apparatus at work. The brain, which looks like a head of cauliflower, grey and squishy to the touch, contains over 15 billion nerve cells, with long fibers of nerve cells linking to other nerve cells in an interweaving jungle of switchboard connections. Messages of sights, sounds, smells, happiness, and pain flash through the connections at breathtaking speed. And in billions of cells are stored memories, emotions, facts, beliefs, reasoning—all the factors that help shape our personalities. Also among those brain cells are the centers that control body functions such as breathing, heartbeat, vision, and speech—as well as waking and sleeping. It's an impressive computer you spend the night with.

The Analysis

In the morning, your electrodes are removed. You then fill out a questionnaire in which you are asked how you felt about the night, how long you thought it took to fall asleep, how many hours you thought you slept, whether it was like sleeping at home, etc. This is to compare what you felt was happening with what the recordings actually show. In some cases, what patients honestly feel and report to their physicians is different from what actually happened. It is important to understand whether you sleep four hours, but feel that you have slept seven hours, or sleep four hours, but feel that you haven't slept at all.

In the morning, sleep specialists also scrutinize the recordings that were made all night. The recording is about 1,000 pages long and weighs about 20 pounds for each patient. Sleep specialists study the summaries and charts that the technicians have put together during the night. They see how long it took you to fall asleep, how long you spent in the different stages of sleep, when you were dreaming and when you were not, whether you snored, when your legs or arms twitched, what your breathing was like, and whether it was correlated with times you woke up. You then have a meeting to talk about the findings—either that morning or at a later time.

About once a month, a patient comes to the clinic who claims not to have slept a wink for months. So far, each has slept more than three hours per night in our sleep lab.

Sam Bush, a 50-year-old janitor, was studied because he claimed that he had't slept a wink for the past five years. He said he rested about six hours a night, but was awake and aware of what was going on at all times. He got up four to six times each night to go to the bathroom, to prepare a snack, or just to walk around. He said that he tossed and turned most of the night. Indeed, because he was so restless, his wife had long since insisted on separate bedrooms. She confirmed that he seemed to be up many times at night, but she also said that occasionally she would hear faint snoring from his room. He adamantly denied ever having slept even a minute for the entire five years.

The tip-off came, however, when Mr. Bush said that he felt well during the day, had enough energy, and felt relatively jovial. Without sleep, this simply is not possible.

We studied him in the lab for three nights. On the first night, we let him lie in bed undisturbed. The polygraph measured about five and a half hours of sleep. He did get up and walk around several times. When asked in the morning how he had slept, he replied, "Not a wink."

On the second night, we called him over the intercom on at least 15 occasions when he was clearly asleep according to the brain waves. Sometimes, we had to call him four or five times before he woke up. However, each time he claimed that he had reacted on the first call and that he had been totally awake.

On the third night, with his permission, we kept him awake all night by talking to him and making him do mental problems while he was in bed. He claimed that this was not any different from what had happened the first two nights and every night at home. However, during the next day, he was extremely tired, irritable, distraught, and even sleepy. Obviously, he had slept quite a lot during the first two nights, but not during the third night.

This patient was not just lying or putting us on. He sincerely believed that he did not sleep. Although we showed him his recording, we could not convince Mr. Bush that he actually slept. Rather, he accused us of slipping him some medication on the third morning that made him so sleepy.

Sometimes this happens. For whatever reasons, some people need to feel that they sleep very little or not at all.

Mystery Patients and Unexplainable Treatments

The one kind of insomnia that is the hardest to help is *primary insomnia,* also called *childhood-onset insomnia.* This is a lifelong inability to obtain adequate sleep and is believed to be caused by an anatomical difference in the nervous system or a chemical imbalance involved with sleep. If one of your first memories as a child is sitting up all night watching the empty street or the rest of the family sleep, you probably have primary insomnia. Also, the insomnia is the same during stress-free periods as in periods of stress.

Studies in our laboratory showed that patients with this type of insomnia take significantly longer to fall asleep than do adult-onset insomniacs, sleep less, and show atypical EEG rhythms, such as periods of REM sleep without eye movements. Their somnograms often are difficult to score, because sleep spindles may be poorly formed and the different sleep stages may be intermixed. These insomniacs often are tremendously sensitive to noise and to stimulants. One cup of tea or some chocolate hours before bedtime may seriously interfere with their sleep.

What can these people do? First, they need to do all the things we have discussed in this book even more thoroughly than anyone else. They need to be scrupulous in getting enough exercise, adhering to rules of sleep hygiene and stress management, staying away from caffeine, and all the other things.

For some reason, sleeping pills usually don't help primary insomnia, but low dosages of antidepressants often do help—dosages that are much too small to be used in depression. Apparently, these antidepressants change some biochemical balances in the brain. Some imbalances can cause insomnia. So, childhood-onset insomnia can sometimes be improved with antidepressants, but it takes trial and error to find the proper one. Patients with primary insomnia usually do not become habituated to low dosages of antidepressants, so they can stay on low dosages for years.

There also seems to be an interrelationship among primary insomnia, dyslexia, and hyperactivity. In a large proportion of primary-insomnia cases, the patient was hyperactive or had dyslexia in childhood. (Dyslexia is an inability to read understandingly because of problems with word perception.) But not all childhood-onset insomniacs were hyperactive or dyslexic, and not all hyperactive children have insomnia. Interestingly, we have found that low dosages of antidepressants occasionally also help in dyslexia and hyperactivity.

Elavil is the one antidepressant that has been studied so far for use in primary insomnia. The adult dosage for clinical depression is about 200 mg; for primary insomnia the dosage is only about 10 to 25 mg. For depression, you have to take the drug for about three weeks before you can tell whether it will help; for insomnia, it works the first or second night if it works at all.

It's too bad that we call these drugs antidepressants, because childhood-onset insomniacs usually are not depressed. In fact, they often cope amazingly well with the condition, when you consider that they have spent most of their lives feeling exhausted and telling doctor after doctor, "I'm not worred about anything, I'm not anxious, I'm not nervous—no, no I'm not." And they are right. In their cases, it is an organic problem.

In addition to Elavil, other antidepressant drugs that cause sedation might work just as well, but they have not been studied yet. So in a person who has side effects from low dosages of Elavil, other antidepressants in low dosages can be tried. You should go to a psychiatrist to determine which antidepressant is best, not because there is an emotional problem in primary insomnia, but because the psychiatrist knows antidepressants best and can come up with the proper dosage and drug combination that will work best for you.

A low dosage of Ritalin (the drug of choice for hyperactive children) has been effective in some patients with primary insomnia. It might be something to try if you were hyperactive as a child and also have had poor sleep since childhood. And there are other medicines that have been useful in some cases.

Carolyn Eggleston, a 40-year-old secretary, had had insomnia as long as she could remember. She happened to be born in the same hospital where the Dartmouth sleep center was located, so her chart could be looked up from the newborn nursery. It said, "This is an unusually alert and happy baby. Every time I come into the nursery, it is alert and awake." The nurse 40 years ago thought this was a good sign, but it was not. The kid simply couldn't sleep.

Miss Eggleston's earliest memories were of nights spent sitting quietly by her window for hours, watching the deserted street below while her parents slept. She remembered grade school as "a constant struggle. I was always tired." In high school, she couldn't drink cola drinks or coffee after lunch because it would keep her up all night. She tried sleeping pills. They helped for a few days or weeks, but none brought lasting relief. Extended evaluations at leading medical centers showed no disorders, except for a general lack of stamina, an emaciated condition, and some signs of possible depression.

In our laboratory, Miss Eggleston slept fitfully for only three or four hours at night. She was easily aroused and, when disturbed, was immediately and fully awake. Most remarkable were her strange sleep patterns: excessive stage 1 sleep; almost no delta sleep; and very poorly defined, irregular sleep spindles that occurred once every five to eight minutes.

Miss Eggleston was given about 40 hours of SMR (sensory motor rhythm) biofeedback training, a very specialized type of feedback that aims to improve the sleep spindles. Her sleep improved somewhat: Lab evaluation showed about 40 minutes more sleep per night, fewer awakenings, and possibly some better-formed sleep spindles. However, her sleep still was not adequate.

She then was placed on 10 mg (later 25 mg) of Elavil at bedtime (a very low dosage). This improved her sleep markedly, and she now has taken this medication for four years. To see if she still needs the medication, once a year she withdraws from it for three weeks—each time with disastrous results.

The efficacy of such low dosages of Elavil remains unexplained and deserves further investigation.

Some insomniacs just don't seem to fit any classification. Sometimes, the problem turns out to be something exotic, such as that they are waking up to escape traumatic dreaming. At other times, we simply can't find what the problem is, and we have to try different things blindly. But every year we learn more, and conditions that we could not cure a few years ago often are now within our grasp.

Blake Alton, a 32-year-old executive, felt that he slept long enough, but his sleep was very shallow. He woke up each morning bone-tired and with stiff muscles. The muscle aches and stiffness disappeared during the morning, but he felt tired all day.

In the laboratory, he slept between seven and eight hours a night. However, throughout NREM sleep, high-amplitude alpha waves continuously intruded into his sleep pattern, making it difficult even to score the record. He was put on a regimen of 50 mg of Elavil at bedtime. He slept more soundly, and the morning stiffness disappeared within a few days. When Elavil lost its effectiveness after some months, he was switched to 50 mg of Thorazine at bedtime, and he has enjoyed good success with this medication over the past two years. But neither Elavil nor Thorazine are indicated for such use, and we still don't understand why they worked.

Then there was Sam Hilliard, a 25-year-old graduate student who had chronic insomnia. Although he claimed that he slept fitfully and for less than five hours a night, his EEG on three consecutive lab nights showed that he had fallen asleep within five minutes each night and had slept throughout his eight hours in bed. Since there didn't seem to be a real problem, no treatment was prescribed.

Shortly after the evaluation, Mr. Hilliard sought help from a therapist who taught him a combination of self-hypnosis, meditation, and relaxation training. The treatment cured his "insomnia"; he claimed that he slept soundly throughout the night. A repeat evaluation in the laboratory showed no change. Sleep, according to the recordings, was excellent both before and after treatment.

Subjectively, there was a dramatic change in Mr. Hilliard's sleep after behavioral treatment. According to the EEG, there was no change. Was there a cure? Was it a placebo effect—did he imagine the improvement? Sleep researchers will disagree on the answer.

Some patients who complain of insomnia turn out to be short sleepers who need little sleep. Other people sleep, but they *dream* that they are awake. One fascinating case was a student who used to get eight hours of sleep every night, but spent all his REM periods dreaming that he was awake, trying to sleep. He was exhausted by morning.

Patients like Mr. Hilliard are labeled "insomnia complaint without objective findings." This means that a convincing and honest complaint of "insomnia," made by an apparently normal person such as Mr. Hilliard, cannot be substantiated with current laboratory procedures. This condition was formerly called *pseudoinsomnia*. However, the important thing to know is that, even though the laboratory findings don't show any change, most of these people say that their sleep improves markedly and they don't feel tired in the morning when they follow the program in this book.

It is possible that some of these patients suffer from a sleep problem whose cause hasn't yet been discovered. There are many sleep disorders that were unknown ten years ago; others will be discovered in the future.

Some patients who have these complaints of poor sleep that defy explanation have tried acupuncture. Some, when traveling in Russia, have tried electrosleep, which is seldom used in America. The treatment consists of giving the patient mild electrical stimulation through electrodes on the eyelids and head for about 15 minutes. We have no experience with either of these treatments.

The Future

The field of research and treatment of sleep disorders is very young. It probably is one of the most exciting new fields in medicine today in terms of the knowledge to be gained and the number of people who can be helped. In fact, there is more research to be done than those of us in sleep research can possibly do in our lifetimes. For example, researchers currently are working on ways to raise the brain's serotonin level or to find a key brain chemical that will produce sleep naturally and provide a natural sleeping pill.

The field of sleep research is growing so quickly that much of what you have learned in this book about sleep was not known ten years ago, not even by physicians or sleep researchers. No doubt, even more people will be able to be helped after another ten years of research. Until then, we wish you the very best of sleep.

Appendix
Sleep Disorders Centers

The following sleep disorders centers are accredited members of the American Sleep Disorders Association. You can obtain a yearly updated list or other information from the American Sleep Disorders Association, 604 2nd St. SW, Rochester, MN 55902. Telephone: 507-287-6006.

Sleep Disorders Centers and Laboratories of the American Sleep Disorders Association

Asterisked centers are accredited specialty laboratories for sleep-related breathing disorders.

Alabama

Sleep Disorders Center of Alabama
Baptist Medical Center Montclair
800 Montclair Road
Birmingham, AL 35213
205-592-5650

Sleep-Wake Disorders Center
University of Alabama
University Station
Birmingham, AL 35294
205-934-7110

Sleep Disorders Laboratory
Children's Hospital of Alabama*
1600 7th Avenue South
Birmingham, AL 35233
205-939-9386

Sleep Disorders Center
Mobile Infirmary Medical Center
P.O. Box 2144
Mobile, AL 36652
205-431-5559

Sleep Disorders Center
Huntsville Hospital
101 Sivley Road
Huntsville, AL 35801
205-533-8553

Arizona

Sleep Disorders Center
Good Samaritan Medical Center
1111 East McDowell Road
Phoenix, AZ 85006
602-239-5815

Sleep Disorders Center
University of Arizona
1501 North Campbell Avenue
Tucson, AZ 85724
602-626-6112

Arkansas

Sleep Disorders Center
Arkansas Children's Hospital
800 Marshall Street
Little Rock, AR 72202-3591
501-370-1893

Sleep Disorders Diagnostic &
    Research Center
University of Arkansas for Medical
    Sciences
4301 West Markham, Slot 594
Little Rock, AR 72205
501-686-6300

Sleep Disorders Center
Baptist Medical Center
9601 1-630, Exit 7
Little Rock, AR 72205-7299
501-227-1902

California

WMCA Sleep Disorders Center
Western Medical Center–Anaheim
1025 South Anaheim Boulevard
Anaheim, CA 92805
714-491-1159

Sleep Disorders Center
Downey Community Hospital
11500 Brookshire Avenue
Downey, CA 90241
213-806-5280

Sleep Disorders Institute
St. Jude Hospital and
    Rehabilitation Center
101 East Valencia Mesa Drive
Fullerton, CA 92634
714-871-3280

Sleep Disorders Center
Scripps Clinic and Research
    Foundation
10666 North Torrey Pines Road
La Jolla, CA 92037
619-554-8087

Sleep Disorders Center
Hospital of the Good Samaritan
616 South Witmer
Los Angeles, CA 90017
213-977-2206

UCLA Sleep Disorders Clinic
Department of Neurology
Room 1155, RNRC
710 Westwood Plaza
Los Angeles, CA 90024
213-206-8005

North Valley Sleep Disorders
    Center
11550 Indian Hills Road, Suite 291
Mission Hills, CA 91345
818-898-4639

Sleep Disorders Center
Hoag Memorial Hospital
    Presbyterian
301 Newport Boulevard
Newport Beach, CA 92663
714-760-2070

Sleep Apnea Center
Merritt-Peralta Medical Center*
450 30th Street
Oakland, CA 94609
415-451-4900

Sleep Disorders Center
U.C. Irvine Medical Center
101 City Drive South
Orange, CA 92668
714-634-5105

Sleep Disorders Center
Huntington Memorial Hospital*
100 Congress Street
Pasadena, CA 91105
818-397-3061

Sleep Disorders Center
Pomona Valley Hospital Medical
    Center
1798 North Garey Avenue
Pomona, CA 91767
714-865-9135

Sleep Disorders Center
Sequoia Hospital
Whipple and Alameda
Redwood City, CA 94062
415-367-5137

Sutter Sleep Disorders Laboratory
Sutter Hospitals*
52nd and F Streets
Sacramento, CA 95819
916-733-1070

San Diego Regional Sleep
    Disorders Center
Harbor View Medical Center and
    Hospital
120 Elm Street
San Diego, CA 92101
619-235-3176

Sleep Disorders Clinic
Stanford University Medical Center
211 Quarry Road, N2A
Stanford, CA 94305
415-723-6601

Southern California Sleep Apnea
    Center
Lombard Medical Group*
2230 Lynn Road
Thousand Oaks, CA 91360
805-495-1066

Sleep Disorders Center
Torrance Memorial Hospital
3330 Lomita Boulevard
Torrance, CA 90509
213-517-4617

Sleep Disorders Center
Kaweah Delta District Hospital*
400 West Mineral King Avenue
Visalia, CA 93291
209-625-7303

Pediatric Sleep Apnea Laboratory
Queen of the Valley Hospital*
1115 South Sunset Avenue
West Covina, CA 91790
818-962-4011

Colorado

Sleep Disorders Center
University of Colorado Health
    Sciences Center
700 Delaware Street
Denver, CO 80204
303-592-7278

National Jewish Center for
    Immunology and Respiratory
    Medicine*
Cardio-Respiratory Sleep Disorders
    Center
1400 Jackson
Denver, CO 80206
303-398-1426

Connecticut

New Haven Sleep Disorders Center
100 York Street
University Towers
New Haven, CT 06511
203-776-9578

District of Columbia

Sleep Disorders Center
Georgetown University Hospital
3800 Reservoir Road, Northwest
Washington, DC 20007-2197
202-784-3610

Florida

Sleep Disorder Laboratory
Broward General Medical Center*
1600 South Andrews Avenue
Fort Lauderdale, FL 33316
305-355-5534

Sleep-Related Breathing Disorders
    Center
Baptist Medical Center*
800 Prudential Drive
Jacksonville, FL 32207
904-674-2909

Center for Sleep Disordered
    Breathing*
P.O. Box 2982
Jacksonville, FL 32203
904-387-7300

Sleep Disorders Center
Mt. Sinai Medical Center
4300 Alton Road
Miami Beach, FL 33140
305-674-2613

Georgia

Sleep Disorders Center
Northside Hospital
1000 Johnson Ferry Road
Atlanta, GA 30342
404-851-8135

Savannah Sleep Disorders Center
Saint Joseph's Hospital
11705 Mercy Boulevard
P.O. Box 60129
Savannah, GA 31420-0129
912-927-5141

Hawaii

Sleep Disorders Center of the
    Pacific
Straub Clinic and Hospital
888 South King Street
Honolulu, HI 96813
808-522-4448

Illinois

Sleep Disorders Center
Rush-Presbyterian-St. Luke's
1753 West Congress Parkway
Chicago, IL 60612
312-942-5440

Sleep Disorders Center
University of Chicago
5841 South Maryland, Box 425
Chicago, IL 60637
312-702-0648

Center for Sleep-Related Breathing
    Disorders
Decatur Memorial Hospital*
2300 North Edward
Decatur, IL 62526
217-877-8121

Sleep Disorders Center
Evanston Hospital
2650 Ridge Avenue
Evanston, IL 60201
708-570-2567

C. Duane Morgan Sleep Disorders
    Center
Methodist Medical Center of
    Illinois
221 Northeast Glen Oak
Peoria, IL 61636
309-672-4966

Carle Regional Sleep Disorders
    Center
602 West University
Urbana, IL 61801
217-337-3364

Indiana

Sleep/Wake Disorders Center
Community Hospitals Indianapolis
1500 North Ritter Avenue
Indianapolis, IN 46219
317-353-4275

Sleep Disorders Center
Winona Memorial Hospital
3232 North Meridian Street
Indianapolis, IN 46208
317-927-2100

Sleep Disorders Center
Lafayette Home Hospital
2400 South Street
Lafayette, IN 47903
317-447-6811

Iowa

Sleep Disorders Center
Mercy Hospital*
West Central Park at Marquette
Davenport, IA 52804
319-383-1071

St. Luke's Sleep Disorders Center
    For Sleep Related Breathing
    Disorders*
1227 East Rusholme Street
Davenport, IA 52803
319-326-6740

Sleep Disorders Center
Iowa Methodist Medical Center
1200 Pleasant Street
Des Moines, IA 50309
515-283-5094

Kentucky

Sleep Disorders Center
St. Joseph's Hospital
One St. Joseph Drive
Lexington, KY 40504
606-278-3436

Sleep Disorders Center
Humana Hospital–Audubon
One Audubon Plaza Drive
Louisville, KY 40217
502-636-7459

Louisiana

Tulane Sleep Disorders Center
1415 Tulane Avenue
New Orleans, LA 70112
504-584-3592

LSU Sleep Disorders Center
Louisiana State University Medical
    Center
P.O. Box 33932
Shreveport, LA 71130-3932
318-674-5365

Maine

Sleep Laboratory
Maine Medical Center*
22 Bramhall Street
Portland, ME 04102
207-871-2279

Maryland

The Johns Hopkins Sleep
    Disorders Center
Francis Scott Key Medical Center
Baltimore, MD 21224
301-550-0571

Maryland Sleep Diagnostic Center
8415 Bellona Lane
Baltimore, MD 21204
301-494-9773

National Capitol Sleep Center
4520 East West Highway
Bethesda, MD 20814
301-656-9515

Massachusetts

Sleep Disorders Unit
Beth Israel Hospital
330 Brookline Avenue, KS430
Boston, MA 02215
617-735-3237

Michigan

Sleep/Wake Disorders Unit
VA Medical Center
Southfield & Outer Drive
Allen Park, MI 48101
313-562-6000

Sleep Disorders Center
University of Michigan Hospitals
1500 East Medical Center Drive
Ann Arbor, MI 48109-0115
313-936-9068

Sleep Disorders Center
Henry Ford Hospital
2799 West Grand Boulevard
Detroit, MI 48202
313-972-1800

Sleep Disorders Program
Ingham Medical Center
401 West Greenlawn Avenue
Lansing, MI 48910-0817
517-334-2510

Sleep Disorders Institute
44199 Dequindre, Suite 403
Troy, MI 48098
313-547-5337

Minnesota

Duluth Regional Sleep Disorders
    Center
St. Mary's Medical Center
407 East Third Street
Duluth, MN 55805
218-726-4692

Sleep Disorders Center
Abbott Northwestern Hospital
800 East 28th Street at Chicago
    Avenue
Minneapolis, MN 55407
612-863-3200

Sleep Disorders Center
Hennepin County Medical Center
701 Park Avenue South
Minneapolis, MN 55415
800-343-6774

Sleep Disorders Center
Mayo Clinic
200 First Street, Southwest
Rochester, MN 55905
507-286-8900

Sleep Disorders Center
Methodist Hospital
6500 Excelsior Boulevard
St. Louis Park, MN 55426
612-932-6083

Mississippi

Sleep Disorders Center
University of Mississippi Medical
    Center
2500 North State Street
Jackson, MS 39216-4505
601-984-4820

Sleep Disorders Center
Memorial Hospital at Gulfport
P.O. Box 1810
Gulfport, MS 39501
601-865-3152 or 865-3495

Missouri

Sleep Disorders Center
Research Medical Center
2316 East Meyer Boulevard
Kansas City, MO 64132-1199
816-276-4222

Sleep Disorders Center
St. Louis University Medical Center
1221 South Grand Boulevard
St. Louis, MO 63104
314-577-8705

Sleep Disorders Center
Deaconess Hospital
6150 Oakland Avenue
St. Louis, MO 63139
314-768-3100

Sleep Disorders Center
L. E. Cox Medical Center
3801 South National Avenue
Springfield, MO 65807
417-885-6189

Nebraska

Sleep Disorders Center
Lutheran Medical Center*
515 South 26th Street
Omaha, NE 68103
402-536-6352

New Hampshire

Sleep-Wake Disorders Center
Hampstead Hospital
East Road
Hampstead, NH 03841
603-329-5311

Dartmouth-Hitchcock Sleep
    Disorders Center
Department of Psychiatry
Dartmouth Medical School
Hanover, NH 03756
603-646-7534

New Jersey

Sleep Disorders Center
Newark Beth Israel Medical Center
201 Lyons Avenue
Newark, NJ 07112
201-926-7163

New York

Sleep-Wake Disorders Center
Montefiore Hospital
111 East 210th Street
Bronx, NY 10467
212-920-4841

Sleep Disorders Center of Western
    New York
Millard Fillmore Hospital
3 Gates Circle
Buffalo, NY 14209
716-884-9253

Sleep Disorders Center
Columbia-Presbyterian Medical
    Center
161 Fort Washington Avenue
New York, NY 10032
212-305-1860

Sleep Disorders Center of
    Rochester
2110 Clinton Avenue South
Rochester, NY 14618
716-442-4141

Sleep Disorders Center
University Hospital
Stony Brook, NY 11794-7139
516-444-2916

The Sleep Center
Community General Hospital
Broad Road
Syracuse, NY 13215

Sleep-Wake Disorders Center
New York Hospital-Cornell
    Medical Center
21 Bloomingdale Road
White Plains, NY 10605
914-997-5751

North Carolina

Sleep Disorders Center
University Memorial Hospital
P.O. Box 560727
W.T. Harris Boulevard at US 29
Charlotte, NC 28256
704-547-9556

North Dakota

Sleep Disorders Center
St. Luke's Hospital
720 4th Street North
Fargo, ND 58122
701-234-5673

Ohio

Sleep Disorders Center
Bethesda Oak Hospital
619 Oak Street
Cincinnati, OH 45206
513-569-6320

The Center for Research in Sleep
   Disorders
Affiliated with Mercy Hospital of
   Hamilton/Fairfield
1275 East Kemper Road
Cincinnati, OH 45246
513-671-3101

Sleep Disorders Center
Department of Neurology
Cleveland Clinic
Cleveland, OH 44106
216-444-2165

Ohio State University
Sleep Disorders Treatment and
   Research Center
473 West 12th Avenue
Columbus, OH 43210
614-293-8296

The Center for Sleep and Wake
   Disorders
Miami Valley Hospital
Thirty Apple Street
Dayton, OH 45409
513-220-2515

Sleep Disorders Center
Kettering Medical Center
3535 Southern Boulevard
Kettering, OH 45429
513-296-7805

Sleep Disorders Center
St. Vincent Medical Center
2213 Cherry Street
Toledo, OH 43608-2691
419-321-4980

Northwest Ohio Sleep Disorders
   Center
The Toledo Hospital
2142 North Cove Boulevard
Toledo, OH 43606
419-471-5629

Oklahoma

Sleep Disorders Center
Presbyterian Hospital
Northeast 13th at Lincoln
   Boulevard
Oklahoma City, OK 73104
405-271-6312

Oregon

Sleep Disorders Center
Rogue Valley Medical Center
2825 Barnett Road
Medford, OR 97504
503-770-4320

Pacific Northwest Sleep Disorders
   Program
Good Samaritan Hospital
1130 Northwest 22nd Avenue
Portland, OR 97210
503-229-8311

Pennsylvania

Sleep Disorders Center
Jefferson Medical College
1015 Walnut Street, Third Floor
Philadelphia, PA 19107
215-928-6175

Sleep Disorders Center
The Medical College of
    Pennsylvania
3200 Henry Avenue
Philadelphia, PA 19129
215-842-4250

Sleep Evaluation Center
Western Psychiatric Institute
3811 O'Hara Street
Pittsburgh, PA 15213-2593
412-624-2246

Sleep Disorders Center
Department of Neurology
Crozer-Chester Medical Center
Upland-Chester, PA 19013
215-447-2689

South Carolina

Sleep Disorders Center
Baptist Medical Center
Taylor at Marion Streets
Columbia, SC 29220
803-771-5557

Children's Sleep Disorders Center
Self Memorial Hospital*
1325 Spring Street
Greenwood, SC 29646
803-227-4449 or 227-4206

Sleep Disorders Center
Spartanburg Regional Medical
    Center
101 East Wood Street
Spartanburg, SC 29303
803-591-6000

South Dakota

Sleep Disorders Center
Sioux Valley Hospital
1100 South Euclid
Sioux Falls, SD 57117-5039
605-333-6302

Tennessee

Sleep Disorders Center
St. Mary's Medical Center
Oak Hill Avenue
Knoxville, TN 37917
615-971-7529

Sleep Disorders Center
Ft. Sanders Regional Medical
    Center
1901 West Clinch Avenue
Knoxville, TN 37916
615-541-1375

BMH Sleep Disorders Center
Baptist Memorial Hospital
899 Madison Avenue
Memphis, TN 38146
901-522-5704

Sleep Disorders Center
Saint Thomas Hospital
Nashville, TN 37202
615-386-2068

Sleep Disorders Center
West Side Hospital
2221 Murphy Avenue
Nashville, TN 37203
615-329-6292

Texas

Sleep-Wake Disorders Center
Presbyterian Hospital
8200 Walnut Hill Lane
Dallas, TX 75231
214-696-8563

Sleep Disorders Center
Sun Towers Hospital
1801 North Oregon
El Paso, TX 79902
915-532-6281

Sleep Disorders Diagnostic and
    Treatment Center
All Saints Episcopal Hospital
1400 8th Avenue
Fort Worth, TX 76104
817-927-6120

Sleep Disorders Center
Baylor College of Medicine
One Baylor Plaza
Houston, TX 77030
713-799-4886

Sleep Disorders Center
Sam Houston Memorial Hospital
8300 Waterbury, Suite 350
Houston, TX 77055
713-973-6483

Sleep Disorders Center
Scott and White Clinic
2401 South 31st Street
Temple TX 76508
817-774-2554

Utah

Sleep Disorders Center
Utah Neurological Clinic
1055 North 300 West, Suite 400
Provo, UT 84604
801-379-7400

Intermountain Sleep Disorders
    Center
LDS Hospital
325 8th Avenue
Salt Lake City, UT 84143
801-321-3417

Virginia

Sleep Disorders Center
Eastern Virginia Medical School
Sentara Norfolk General Hospital
600 Gresham Drive
Norfolk, VA 23507
804-628-3322

Medical College of Virginia Sleep
    Disorders Center
Medical College of Virginia
P.O. Box 710-MCV Station
Richmond, VA 23298
804-786-1993

Sleep Disorders Center
Community Hospital of Roanoke
    Valley
P.O. Box 12946
Roanoke, VA 24029
703-985-8435

Washington

Sleep Disorders Center
Providence Medical Center
500 17th Avenue, C-34008
Seattle, WA 98124
206-326-5366

Sacred Heart Sleep Apnea Center
Sacred Heart Medical Center*
West 101 Eighth Avenue, TAF C9
Spokane, WA 99220-4045
509-455-4895

Wisconsin

Wisconsin Sleep Disorders Center
Gundersen Clinic
1836 South Avenue
La Crosse, WI 54601
608-782-7300

Sleep/Wake Disorders Center
St. Mary's Hospital
2323 North Lake Drive
Milwaukee, WI 53201-0503
414-225-8032

Milwaukee Regional Sleep
    Disorders Center
Columbia Hospital
2025 East Newport Avenue
Milwaukee, WI 53211
414-961-4650

Sleep Disorders Centers in Canada

For information about sleep disorders centers in Canada, you may contact the following:

Harvey Moldofsky M.D.
Canadian Sleep Society
Sleep Disorders Clinic
Western Division, Toronto Hospital
399 Bathurst Street
Toronto M5T258 Ontario
Canada

Sleep Disorders Centers in Latin America

For information about sleep disorders centers in Latin America, you may contact the following:

Rubens Reimao M.D.
Latinamerican Sleep Society
Rua Glicineas 128
04048 São Paulo, SP
Brazil
Phone: 55 011 845-1233
Fax: 55 011 842-2834

Sleep Disorders Centers in Europe

For information about sleep disorders centers in Europe, you may contact the following:

Dr. Dag Stenberg
Department of Physiology
Siltavuorenpenger 20J
SF-00170 Helsinki
Finland

Sleep Disorders Centers in Japan

For information about sleep disorders centers in Japan, you may contact the following:

Kazuo Azumi M.D.
Japanese Sleep Research Society
Psychophysiology of Sleep
Tokyo Metropolitan Institute for Neurosciences
2-6 Musashi-Dai
Fuchu City, Tokyo 183
Japan

Sleep Disorders Centers in Australia and Nearby Areas

For information about sleep disorders centers in Australia and nearby areas, you may contact the following:

Leon Lack Ph.D.
Australasian Sleep Research Association
Psychology Discipline
Flinders University
Bedford Park, South Australia
5042 Australia

Glossary

A

ACUTE—A term applied to short, severe attacks of a disease or of pain.

ALPHA-DELTA SLEEP—A type of sleep during which the EEG shows a mixture of alpha (awake) and NREM (asleep) waves. Alpha-delta sleep is nonrestorative, leading to malaise upon awakening.

ALPHA RHYTHM—A brain wave pattern seen in relaxed wakefulness, characterized by 8- to 12-cycle-per-second EEG waves.

ANTIDEPRESSANT—Anything that counteracts clinical depression.

ANTIHISTAMINE—A drug used to counter the effects of histamine, a chemical produced by the body as a result of an inflammatory and allergic reaction. Used in some nonprescription sleeping pills.

ANXIETY—A feeling of apprehension.

APNEA—A pause in breathing that lasts ten seconds or longer. A person with the sleep-apnea syndrome has many apneas during sleep.

AROUSAL—*Partial arousal* is a change from a deep stage of NREM sleep to a lighter one. *Full arousal* means awakening. During an arousal, your EEG changes, your muscle tone increases, your heart beats faster, and you may move.

AUTOMATIC BEHAVIOR—A type of behavior that is carried out without the person being conscious of it.

AUTONOMIC NERVOUS SYSTEM—The part of the nervous system that innervates smooth and cardiac muscle and glandular tissues and governs involuntary action.

AWAKE—A state in which brain waves are of the alpha or beta patterns; also known as a fast EEG. The person is conscious and aware of the surroundings.

B

BASAL METABOLISM—The lowest possible metabolic rate in the body resulting in the lowest body temperature; usually, the lowest is about one hour before rising.

BETA WAVES—Usually associated with alert wakefulness. They are faster than alpha waves, cycling about 13 to 35 times per second.

BIOFEEDBACK—A technique using instrumentation to provide moment-to-moment information about body processes that a person normally is not aware of, so that he or she can learn to control them. It may be used to teach a person to regulate muscle tension, heart rate, blood pressure, blood flow, skin temperature, and the activity of the gastrointestinal tract, among other processes.

BOOTZIN TECHNIQUE—Also called stimulus-control therapy. A treatment for conditioned insomnia in which the patient is asked to get out of bed if he or she cannot fall asleep easily.

BRAINSTEM—The part of the nervous system located at the base of the brain, connecting the spinal cord with the rest of the brain; it is thought to contain all the mechanisms necessary for survival, including the mechanisms that regulate sleep-waking behavior.

BRAIN-WAVE RHYTHMS—Patterns of electrical activity of the brain.

C

CATAPLEXY—A sudden attack of complete or partial muscular paralysis, usually precipitated by a strong emotion. Cataplexy usually is a symptom of narcolepsy.

CHRONIC—A condition that has lasted, or is expected to last, for quite some time.

CHRONOBIOLOGY—The science of rhythmic functions in living things.

CHRONOTHERAPY—A treatment technique for the delayed-sleep-phase syndrome. The patient is asked to go to bed each night three hours later, until his or her bedtime equals the desired bedtime.

CIRCADIAN RHYTHM—An innate, daily fluctuation of physiological and behavioral functions, including sleep and waking; generally tied to the 24-hour light-and-dark day-night cycle. The innate periodicity usually is not exactly 24 hours; hence, the prefix *circa* (meaning *about*).

COGNITIVE THERAPY—A form of psychotherapy based on the idea that a person's emotional responses are influenced by what he or she thinks. The therapist works with the patient to change any maladaptive patterns of thinking.

CONDITIONED INSOMNIA—An easily overlooked form of chronic insomnia caused by the development, during an earlier experience of sleeplessness, of a negative association between characteristics of the customary sleep environment and sleeping.

D

DELTA SLEEP—The time of deep sleep marked by large, slow EEG, waves, called delta waves, when most bodily recovery is believed to occur. Delta sleep includes both sleep stages 3 and 4. Most delta sleep occurs during the first 90 minutes of sleep. The amount decreases with age. The longer one sleeps, the *less* delta sleep one gets.

DELTA WAVES—EEG waves occurring chiefly in delta sleep; also known as sleep stages 3 and 4 or slow-wave sleep. Delta waves cycle 1/2 to 2 times per second.

DEPRESSANT—Any drug that decreases functional activity; for example, a central-nervous-system depressant is a drug that slows activity in the central-nervous-system.

DYSSOMNIA—A disorder involving the amount and/or timing of sleep, such as insomnia, excessive daytime sleepiness, or circadian-rhythm disturbances.

E

ELECTROENCEPHALOGRAM (EEG)—A recording of the electrical activity of the brain, using a procedure called electroencephalography. It involves placing metal tabs on the head, amplifying the current, and displaying it graphically.

ELECTROMYOGRAM (EMG)—A recording of electrical activity from the muscular system. Electrodes are used to measure activity from the chin muscles and from the legs to assess periodic leg movements, and sometimes from the chest, to assess its movements.

ELECTRO-OCULOGRAM (EOG)—A recording of electrical changes resulting from shifts in position of the eyeball; along with the EEG and the EMG, it is one of the three basic variables used to score sleep stages and waking. It uses surface electrodes placed near the eyes to record the movement of the eyeballs. Rapid eye movements in sleep indicate the REM (dreaming) stage of sleep.

EXCESSIVE DAYTIME SOMNOLENCE (Sleepiness)—Difficulty in staying awake, even after apparently adequate sleep.

F

FIRST-NIGHT EFFECT—The finding that many people do not sleep as well on the first night in a sleep lab as they do later. Some insomniacs display a reverse first-night effect, sleeping best during the first lab night.

FREE-RUNNING—A term in chronobiology indicating that a person's internal rhythm is not being synchronized with the cycle of the sun. Occurs when people are put into time-free environments.

H

HALF-LIFE—The time it takes for one-half of a drug to be eliminated from the body by excretion or metabolism.

HYPERSOMNIA—Excessive or prolonged sleep.

HYPNAGOGIC—Occurring at the beginning of sleep.

HYPNAGOGIC IMAGES—Vivid images that occur at the beginning of sleep. These are particularly intense when sleep begins with a REM period, as frequently occurs in narcolepsy. Such images also may occur just before awakening; these are called *hypnopompic* images.

HYPNAGOGIC JERK—A startle reaction; a harmless sudden body jerk that many persons experience just as sleep begins.

HYPNOPOMPIC—Occurring at the end of sleep, during the process of awakening.

HYPNOPOMPIC HALLUCINATION—An image or a sound in a momentary dream as you wake up.

HYPNOTIC—Related to sleep. The term also is used as a synonym for sleeping pills.

I

IDIOPATHIC INSOMNIA—Insomnia without known cause.

INSOMNIA—The inability to get as much sleep as a person needs for efficient daytime functioning. Literally means *no sleep*, although all insomniacs do get some sleep each 24-hour period.

INTERNAL AROUSAL INSOMNIA—A form of chronic insomnia resulting from excessive mental activity; induced by too-conscious efforts to sleep and underlying apprehension that all attempts will fail.

J

JET-LAG SYNDROME—A maladjustment experienced when an abrupt change in the length of a day causes "body time" or circadian rhythm to be out of phase temporarily with local clock time.

L

LIGHT SLEEP—A term often used for sleep stages 1 and 2.

LONG SLEEPER—A person who usually sleeps more than nine hours, without there being anything wrong with his or her sleep.

M

METABOLISM—A general term designating all chemical changes that occur within the body. Any body reaction may be described as metabolic. Also refers to the body process concerned with the breakdown of food and its use by the cells, including the input and output of energy, heat, and wastes from a cell as it functions.

MINISLEEP—A lapse from wakefulness into sleep that lasts just a few seconds; often associated with excessive daytime sleepiness and automatic behavior.

MULTIPLE SLEEP LATENCY TEST (MSLT)—A test to measure how sleepy you are by observing how long it takes you to fall asleep during your normal waking hours. It is given at least four times in one day at two-hour intervals and is used to diagnose various sleep disorders and to evaluate sleeping pills.

MYOCLONUS—A muscle contraction that produces a jerk or twitch. Often refers to the periodic limb movements that occur in some sleepers.

N

NARCOLEPSY—A neurological disorder that causes irresistible sleepiness.

NEONATAL SLEEP—Pertaining to the sleep of infants in the first four weeks after birth.

NEURO-—Pertaining to the body's nervous system. For example, a *neurologist* is a doctor who specializes in treating diseases of the brain and the nervous system.

NOCTURNAL CONFUSION—Episodes of disorientation close to or during nighttime sleep; often seen in the elderly and indicative of central nervous system deterioration; often referred to as the *sundowner's syndrome.*

NOCTURNAL PENILE TUMESCENCE (NPT) TEST—Assessment during sleep of erections of the penis that occur during REM sleep in healthy males of all ages. Documenting the presence or absence of erections aids in the diagnosis of impotence.

NONRESTORATIVE SLEEP—Also called alpha-delta sleep. Sleep that is not refreshing. During nonrestorative sleep, there is a mixture of alpha and NREM sleep waves, instead of the usual pattern of sleep waves.

NREM SLEEP (Pronounced Non-Rem)—Non-rapid-eye-movement sleep; that is, all the sleep except for REM sleep. NREM and REM periods alternate during sleep in cycles that last approximately 90 minutes. NREM sleep includes stages 1, 2, 3, and 4.

P

PARASOMNIA—A disturbance that occurs during sleep, such as a nightmare, bed-wetting, or sleepwalking.

PAVOR NOCTURNIS—Sleep terrors or night terrors that occur almost exclusively in children. Episodes of this sleep disorder usually arise from the depths of the first stage 4 sleep of night and generally are associated with intense body movements.

PERIODIC LIMB MOVEMENTS—Repetitive twitching, usually of the legs and feet, during sleep. Leg jerks occur in regular intervals 10 to 60 seconds apart and may or may not wake the sleeper.

PHASE ADVANCE—The movement to a position earlier in the 24-hour sleep-wake cycle of a period of sleep or wakefulness; for example, a change of sleeping from 11 P.M. to 7 A.M. to sleeping from 8 P.M. to 4 A.M. Often seen in the elderly.

PHASE DELAY—The opposite of phase advance; that is, a shift to a later sleep time—for example, a change of sleeping from 11 P.M. to 6 A.M. to sleeping from 3 to 10 A.M. Often seen in 15- to 25-year-olds.

PHOTOTHERAPY—The treatment of circadian rhythm disturbances with bright lights (usually more than 2,500 lux).

PLACEBO—An inert substance sometimes given to a research group of patients as part of a drug study. Patients are said to exhibit the *placebo effect* when their health status improves despite the fact that the substance they are taking has no active ingredient.

POLYGRAPH—An instrument for simultaneously recording tracings of several different physiological variables.

POLYSOMNOGRAM—The continuous and simultaneous recording of physiological variables during sleep. The three basic activities that are measured are brain waves, eye movements, and chin-muscle activity; breathing, heart rate, and other functions often are recorded also.

PONS—A part of the brainstem lying between the medulla oblongata and the mesencephalon. The pons is one of the most important parts of the brain with regard to sleep and wakefulness, especially the switching between REM and NREM sleep.

PSEUDOINSOMNIA—Now called *insomnia complaint without objective findings*. The complaint of disturbed sleep despite essentially normal sleep patterns in sleep recordings.

R

REBOUND INSOMNIA—Disrupted sleep that may occur for a few nights after a person stops taking sleeping pills.

REM BEHAVIOR DISORDER—A parasomnia during which the patient carries out part of his or her dreams. It is thought to be due to malfunctioning in those brainstem nuclei that are supposed to inhibit all muscle tone during REM sleep.

REM REBOUND or RECOVERY—An increased amount of REM sleep for a few nights after a period of REM deprivation. REM rebound may occur after one or more nights without REM sleep, or upon withdrawal from certain pills that suppress REM sleep. Increased amounts of REM sleep may be reflected by disturbing dreams.

REM SLEEP—Named for the rapid eye movements that typically occur during this time. It is a period of intense brain activity, often associated with dreams. There is a paralysis of voluntary muscles. REM sleep usually represents about 20 to 25 percent of total sleep time in a young adult. In humans, REM sleep occurs regularly about every 90 minutes.

RIP VAN WINKLE SYNDROME—Becoming groggy and less alert if you sleep too long in the morning.

S

SAWTOOTH WAVES—Waveforms seen uniquely in the EEGs of humans during REM periods. They tend to occur in bursts of two to five waves at a rate of four to seven waves per second and often precede or overlap a burst of rapid eye movement. They are a form of theta waves.

SEROTONIN—A naturally occurring neurotransmitter involved mainly in inhibiting nerve cell activity. The compound is manufactured from tryptophan.

SHORT SLEEPER—A person who usually sleeps less than five hours, without there being anything wrong with his or her sleep.

SLEEP CYCLE—Typically, NREM and REM sleep alternate through the night. The first sleep cycle lasts from sleep onset to the end of the first REM period; the second sleep cycle is measured from the end of the first REM period to the end of the second REM period; and so forth. When all cycles are totaled and averaged, their mean value is near 90 minutes for young adults.

SLEEP EFFICIENCY—The ratio of total sleep time to time in bed. If you stay in bed for eight hours, but sleep only six hours, your sleep efficiency is 75 percent.

SLEEP HYGIENE—The conditions and practices that promote effective sleep. These include regularity of bedtime and arise time, restriction of alcohol and caffeine before bedtime, exercise, proper bedroom environment, and other factors.

SLEEPING SICKNESS—A brain inflammation that occurs in people living in Africa. It is caused by a parasite transmitted to humans by the tsetse fly. The parasites first cause a fever, then enter the central nervous system and cause encephalitis, which results in extreme lethargy and a sleepy appearance.

SLEEP LATENCY—The time from lights-out until the beginning of sleep.

SLEEP LOG—A daily, written record of an individual's sleep-wake pattern containing such information as time of retiring and arising, time in bed, estimated total sleep period, number and duration of sleep interruptions, quality of sleep, daytime naps. An accompanying Day Log is kept to record the use of caffeine, waking activities, and other data.

SLEEP MENTATION—Images and thoughts experienced during sleep. Imagery is vividly expressed in dreams during REM sleep; in NREM sleep, there usually is only short and fragmented thinking.

SLEEP PARALYSIS—An inability to move voluntarily, occurring just at the beginning of sleep or on awakening; may last from a few seconds to a few minutes. Sleep-onset paralysis usually is related to narcolepsy; paralysis at the end of sleep may be scary, but is not clinically significant and frequently occurs in healthy people.

SLEEP SPINDLE—A typical waveform seen in EEGs during NREM sleep and characterized by a burst of very regular oscillations at a frequency of 12 to 14 cycles per second. Sleep spindles are observed most often during NREM EEG stage 2, but they also may be seen in stages 3 and 4.

SOMNOLOGIST—A specialist in the study of sleep and in the diagnosis and treatment of sleep disorders.

STIMULUS-CONTROL THERAPY—See Bootzin technique.

SYMPATHETIC NERVOUS SYSTEM—The part of the nervous system that causes the emergency reaction (fight or flight) with speeding heartbeat, dilating pupils of the eyes, increased blood pressure, etc.

T

THETA WAVES—Brain-wave activity with a frequency of 4 to 8 cycles per second, typically found in light sleep (stages 1 and 2) and in REM sleep.

TWITCH—A very small body movement such as a facial grimace or leg jerk.

U

UPTAKE—The time it takes for a drug to become active after ingestion.

W

WAKE AFTER SLEEP ONSET (WASO)—The amount of time you are awake during the night after you initially fell asleep.

Z

ZEITGEBER—Literally, *time-giver*. An environmental time cue (such as light) that helps to entrain the body's rhythm to the 24-hour day.

ZZZZs—What we want you to get plenty of, in peace and tranquility, after reading this book and following our program. We wish you many happy ZZZZs.

Index

About the Authors

Peter Hauri, **PhD**, is Director of the Mayo Clinic Insomnia Program and co-director of the Sleep Disorders Center at the Mayo Clinic. Born in Switzerland, but living in the US since 1960, he was, for many years, director of the Dartmouth Sleep Disorders Center and on the faculty of Dartmouth Medical School. Considered by many as the world's leading authority on insomnia, Dr. Hauri is the author of *The Sleep Disorders*—a classic for physicians and with half a million copies sold, the most widely read publication in the history of sleep medicine. A pioneer in sleep research, he set up one of the first clinical sleep disorders centers in the US, and was a founder of the American Sleep Disorders Association.

Shirley Linde, **PhD**, is a bestselling author and coauthor of 24 books, including *Dr. Atkins Superenergy Diet Book*, and numerous articles on science, health, and medical issues. She has been an officer of the National Association of Science Writers and the American Medical Writers Association, and is a member of the American Society of Journalists and Authors. A recipient of the Outstanding Service Award from the American Medical Writers Association, as well as the Communicaions Award from Brandeis University. Dr. Linde is listed in Who's Who in America, The World's Who's Who of Women, and Foremost Women of the Twentieth Century.